KT-178-438

Skills for Communicating with Patients

Withdrawn from
√back 16/4/24

Jonathan Silverman
Suzanne Kurtz
and
Juliet Draper

Forewords by

Barbara Korsch
Professor of Pediatrics
University of Southern California
School of Medicine

and

Sir David Weatherall
Regius Professor of Medicine
University of Oxford

Cefn Coed Library
Z001265

LIBRARY
SWANSEA PSYCHIATRIC EDUCATION CENTRE
THE CHURCH
CEFN COED HOSPITAL
COCKETT
SWANSEA SA2 0GH

Radcliffe Medical Press

© 1998 Jonathan Silverman, Suzanne Kurtz and Juliet Draper

Radcliffe Medical Press Ltd
18 Marcham Road, Abingdon, Oxon OX14 1AA, UK

Reprinted 1999

All rights reserved. No part of this publication may be reproduced, stored in a retrieval system, or transmitted, in any form or by any means, electronic, mechanical, photocopying, recording or otherwise without the prior permission of the copyright owner.

British Library Cataloguing in Publication Data

A catalogue record for this book is available from the British Library.

ISBN 1 85775 189 2

Typeset by Advance Typesetting Ltd, Oxon
Printed and bound in Great Britain by Bookcraft (Bath) Ltd.

Contents

Forewords   v
Preface   ix
About this book   xi
About the authors   xiii
Acknowledgements   xv
Introduction   xvii

1   **Defining what to teach and learn: an overview of the communication
    skills curriculum**   1
    Introduction
    Plan of chapter
    Defining the broad types of communication skills
    An overall curriculum of skills: the *Calgary–Cambridge observation guide*
    The need for a structure
    Choosing the skills to include in the communication curriculum
    Skills and individuality
    Issue-specific skills
    Summary

2   **Initiating the session**   17
    Introduction
    Problems in communication
    Objectives
    Skills
    'What' to teach and learn about the initiation – the evidence for the skills
       Preparation
       Establishing initial rapport
       Identifying the reason(s) for the consultation
    Summary

3   **Gathering information**   35
    Introduction
    Problems in communication

A theoretical discussion of information gathering
Objectives
'What' to teach and learn about gathering information – the evidence for the skills
    Section 1: Exploration of problems
    Section 2: Understanding the patient's perspective
    Section 3: Providing structure to the consultation
Summary

4   **Building the relationship**   **71**
Introduction
Problems in communication
Objectives
'What' to teach and learn about the relationship – the evidence for the skills
    Section 1: Non-verbal communication
    Section 2: Developing rapport
    Section 3: Involving the patient
Summary

5   **Explanation and planning**   **89**
Introduction
Problems in communication
Objectives
'What' to teach and learn about explanation and planning – the evidence for the skills
    Section 1: Providing the correct amount and type of information
    Section 2: Aiding accurate recall and understanding
    Section 3: Achieving a shared understanding: incorporating the patient's perspective
    Section 4: Planning – shared decision making
    Section 5: Options in explanation and planning
Summary: explanation and planning is an interactive collaborative process

6   **Closing the session**   **129**
Introduction
Objectives
'What' to teach and learn about endings – the evidence for the skills
Summary

7   **Relating specific issues to core communication skills**   **135**
Introduction
Specific issues
Other specific issues, contexts and challenges
Further reading

References   149

Index   161
Author index   171

Foreword

These two texts on teaching and learning the skills of medical communication are a most welcome addition to the all too sparsely available literature on a topic which is now acknowledged to be crucial in the education and practice of all practitioners, and which is especially important for educators in the health professions. Together, these two books represent one more giant step forward in the evolution of our understanding of the patient–physician relationship and of communication skills in medicine.

What used to be considered the 'art' of medicine, a matter of intuition and personal attributes and hence unresearchable and certainly unteachable, has transmuted into a respectable field of science which is increasingly included explicitly in medical and related curricula. In spite of this evolution there has been a lack of data-based comprehensive literature on the subject. There is an impressive body of research and a large number of publications in the field of patient–clinician communication as such, but for the educator who needs to organize a curriculum, or even a single course, there has been little resource. Even though more institutions recognize the need for teaching this aspect of health care, there is a universal lack of trained faculty, and a deplorable lack of formalized credible documentation of sound principles for teaching this challenging subject. This lack makes it cumbersome for educators to formulate their teaching programme, as well as posing an additional barrier in the ever-continuing battle for a 'place in the sun', i.e. time in the curriculum to teach the doctor–patient relationship and related communication skills.

'What exactly is it that you want to teach?' is a question with which I have been challenged throughout my career. The text by Kurtz, Silverman and Draper contains the answer to this query. In a clear, concise but comprehensive manner the authors tell not only what, but also how and why communication skills should be learned and taught.

In this foreword there is no need to provide a detailed description of the two books' contents, the authors have done so very effectively in their introduction. I do want to underline one feature of the work that is of fundamental importance, namely that the material presented is carefully documented from available research. Data from the communication literature, including the important recent work relating not only outcomes such as patient satisfaction and compliance but also biological and functional patient outcomes to communication variables, are appropriately cited. In their presentation, the authors also bring together the growing body of evidence on the effectiveness of teaching about the doctor–patient relationship, and the duration of the desirable behaviour changes in the learner that can be achieved. Here again the authors provide valuable ammunition to the courageous proponents of teaching communication when challenged by their colleagues dealing with 'hard science' who consistently demand evidence for the value of this kind of teaching, even though the traditional aspects of medical education are frequently not submitted to this rigorous scrutiny.

The whole work is based on the principles for effective adult education. This is especially welcome because medical education, perhaps partly in light of the unfortunate tradition of considering the development of medical professionals as 'training' rather than education, is frequently not sufficiently learner-oriented. This in turn may contribute to clinicians' reluctance later in their practise to make their interactions sufficiently patient-centred. Thus this work, addressed to both learners and teachers, models the kind of communication that is being advocated.

Another welcome contribution is the emphasis on the integration and timing of communication teaching into the entire medical education programme instead of relegating the subject to one isolated course early in the curriculum, which may not even be a requirement, for which the students may not receive formal evaluation, which is considered a luxury not an essential, and which is the first to be cut when there is lack of time in the curriculum or when there is a fiscal exigency.

This work presents significant progress in the field of medical education at a time when there are dramatic changes in medical practice which make communication teaching mandatory and urgent.

Barbara Korsch
January 1998

Foreword

When these two extensive works on communication skills arrived on my desk I was reminded of that fine poem by John Dunne, *The Good Morrow,* in which he asks his lover whether there was any real existence before they met: 'Were we not weaned 'til then, But supped on country pleasures, childishly? Or snorted we in the seven sleepers' den?' As judged by recent attacks from all sides on its lack of ability to communicate, not to mention the rediscovery of 'evidence-based medicine', it appears that the medical profession has snorted happily for many centuries, or at least since the advent of high-technology practice and managed health care left it with neither the inclination nor time to sit down and talk to its patients.

While I suspect that at least a few physicians of the past must have been competent communicators, and it is only necessary to read of the life and work of Thomas Sydenham to realize that this must have been the case, it is certainly true that an awareness of the central role of fostering communication skills in medical education and clinical practice is a fairly recent phenomenon. During my time as a medical student in the 1950s, with the possible exception of developing a systemized approach to history taking, the subject was rarely mentioned. Rather, we were expected to learn how to interact with patients by osmosis, sitting dutifully hour after hour in outpatient departments watching the great men at work. I still vividly remember my first ward round with one of the most distinguished physicians in my teaching centre. We arrived at the bedside of a patient who had just been diagnosed as having carcinoma of the bronchus. We suddenly veered away from the bedside, formed a rugby scrum in the middle of the ward, whispered dire prognostications, returned briefly to the patient to utter a few meaningless banalities, and moved on. I have no idea who told that patient about the nature of his illness, if, indeed, anybody ever did. If bad news had to be broken, and so often it did, it was invariably left to the junior staff, who usually asked medical students to leave the room. I don't recall ever sitting in on a discussion about a terminal illness with a patient or their family. Overall, I suspect, we went out into the hard world totally unprepared for applying what is clearly the most important of all the clinical skills.

As will be plain to anybody who delves into these two excellent books, all this has changed. There is a growing awareness that communication is, together with an ability to listen, the most important aspect of practice that students and young (and not so young) doctors have to master. Modern high-technology diagnostic aids have not altered this fact. Indeed, with our increasingly ageing population and the extraordinarily complex ways in which diseases present and are forged by patients' lifestyles and environments, an ability to talk to our patients is becoming even more important. If the growing attractiveness of complementary medicine is telling us anything, it is that conventional western practice is losing its pastoral skills, particularly those which require both the time and ability to comfort sick people and their families.

Although it happens more often as one becomes a geriatric statistic, there is still no happier surprise and compliment than to be invited to write a foreword to a book by one of one's ex-students. In this case it is a particular pleasure because the subject is so important and central to many of the problems of the current clinical scene. What is even more encouraging to somebody who has tried, with limited success, to impress the importance of the scientific basis of medicine on young people is, as witnessed by these books, that considerable efforts are being made to try to measure the outcome of new approaches to teaching the skills of communication.

I hope that *all* those involved in medical education, and not a few students and doctors of all ages, will browse through these pages, lie in the bath and mull over what they have read, and then go straight to their wards, outpatients or practices and start really talking to sick people. While no amount of reading or teaching can make up for communicating directly with patients and their friends and families, and learning from one's mistakes over a lifetime, the modern approaches to improving this skill, so well presented in these books, are providing an increasingly valuable basis on which to build the most important of all the attributes that make for a good doctor.

David Weatherall
January 1998

Preface

Skills for Communicating with Patients is one of a set of two companion books on improving communication in medicine which together provide a comprehensive approach to teaching and learning communication throughout all three levels of medical education (undergraduate, residency and continuing medical education) and in both specialist and family medicine.

In our first book, *Teaching and Learning Communication Skills in Medicine*, we examine how to construct a communication skills curriculum, document the individual skills that form the core content of communication skills teaching programmes and explore in depth the specific teaching and learning methods employed in this unique field of medical education. Our first book presents:

- an overall rationale for communication skills teaching – the 'why', the 'what' and the 'how' of teaching and learning communication skills in medicine
- the individual skills that constitute effective doctor–patient communication
- a systematic approach for presenting, learning and using these skills in practice
- a detailed description of appropriate teaching and learning methods, including:
  - innovative approaches to analysis and feedback in experiential teaching sessions
  - key facilitation skills that maximize participation and learning
- principles, concepts and research evidence that substantiate the specific teaching and learning methods used in communication skills programmes
- strategies for constructing a communication skills curriculum in practice.

This second book, *Skills for Communicating with Patients*, undertakes a more detailed exploration of the specific skills of doctor–patient communication. We not only examine how to use these skills in the medical interview but also provide comprehensive evidence of the improvements that communication skills can make to both everyday clinical practice and to ensuing health outcomes. This book presents:

- the individual skills that form the core content of communication skills teaching programmes
- an overall structure which helps organize the skills and our teaching and learning about them
- a detailed description and rationale for the use of each of these core skills in the medical interview

- principles, concepts and research evidence that validate the importance of the skills and document the potential gains for doctors and patients alike
- suggestions for how to use each skill in practice
- a discussion of the major role that these core communication skills play in dealing with specific communication issues and challenges.

We encourage our readers to study both books. While at first glance, it would appear that this volume might be exclusively for learners and our companion volume exclusively for teachers, this is far from our intention:

- facilitators need as much help with 'what' to teach as 'how' to teach. We demonstrate how in-depth knowledge of the use of communication skills and of the accompanying research evidence is essential if facilitators wish to maximize learning in their experiential teaching sessions
- learners need to understand 'how' to learn as well as 'what' to learn. Understanding the principles of communication skills teaching will enable learners to maximize their own learning throughout the communication curriculum, improve their own participation in that learning, understand the value of observation and rehearsal, provide constructive feedback and contribute to the formation of a supportive climate.

In communication skills teaching there is a fine line between teachers and learners. Teachers will continue to make discoveries about communication throughout their professional lives and learn from their students. Learners not only teach their peers but soon become the communication skills teachers of the next generation of doctors, whether formally, informally or as role-models. No doctor can escape this responsibility.

Jonathan Silverman
Suzanne Kurtz
Juliet Draper
January 1998

About this book

This book and its companion work are the result of a happy and fruitful collaboration between the three authors. It began with Dr Silverman taking a sabbatical with Professor Kurtz at the Faculty of Medicine, University of Calgary, Canada in 1993. Professor Kurtz and her colleagues have been developing and implementing communication curricula in medicine, as well as methods for improving communication in other areas of health care, since the mid 1970s. Dr Silverman and Dr Draper have been working together to run communication skills teaching in postgraduate general practice in the East Anglian Region of the UK since 1989. Over the past four years the collaboration between the three authors has led to a cross-fertilization of ideas and methods and resulted in the writing of these books.

Professor Kurtz and Dr Silverman share first authorship equally for both titles and to reflect this equality Professor Kurtz is listed as first author for *Teaching and Learning Communication Skills in Medicine* and Dr Silverman is listed as first author for *Skills for Communicating with Patients*.

About the authors

Dr Suzanne M Kurtz, PhD is Professor of Communication in the Faculties of Education and Medicine of the University of Calgary, Canada. Focusing her career on improving communication and educational practices in health care and education, development of communication curricula, and clinical skills evaluation, she has worked with medical and education students, residents, practising physicians, nurses, allied health professionals, patient groups, teachers and administrators. For over 20 years she has co-directed the undergraduate communication curriculum in Calgary's Faculty of Medicine and is called on nationally and internationally at all levels of medical education for her expertise in the specifics of setting up effective communication programmes. Working across diverse cultural and disciplinary lines, she has also collaborated on several international development projects related to health and education in Nepal, Southeast Asia, and Zululand. Her publications include an earlier book co-authored with VM Riccardi and entitled *Communication and counselling in health care* (Charles C Thomas 1983).

Dr Jonathan Silverman, FRCGP is a general practitioner in Linton, Cambridgeshire, and Communication Skills Teaching Facilitator for Postgraduate General Practice in the Regional General Practice Office of the Anglia and Oxford Regional Health Authority. He has been a trainer for 10 years and was a course organizer of the Cambridge Vocational Training Scheme for five years. For the last eight years he has been organizer of the facilitator training programmes in general practice communication skills in East Anglia. In 1993, he was on sabbatical for six months with the aid of BMA, RCGP and ACO travelling fellowships working with Suzanne Kurtz, teaching and researching communication skills at the Faculty of Medicine, University of Calgary. He is presently developing a module in communication skills for the Masters Degree in Primary and Community Care at the University of Cambridge.

Dr Juliet Draper, FRCGP, MD is a general practitioner in Cambridge and course organizer of the Cambridge Vocational Training Scheme. She is a trainer in general practice and organizer and evaluator of the facilitator training programmes in general practice communication skills in East Anglia. She has an MD in community antenatal care and has published on health visiting, consumer views on antenatal care and HRT. She has a particular interest in counselling in medical settings and has been involved in the development of the attachment of counsellors in primary care.

Acknowledgements

This book would not have been written without the help of patients, learners and colleagues from all over the world. They have taught us so much and we owe them a great debt.

Many people have helped us directly and indirectly with their ideas, support and time, in particular our families and the people we work with regularly – the preceptors and trainers in our courses, our partnerships and the secretaries, actors and audio-visual technicians who assist us.

We want especially to acknowledge Catherine Heaton, MD for her creative work and continuous support over the past 15 years as co-director and co-author of the undergraduate communication curriculum in Calgary. Her substantive professional contributions to the teaching and evaluation programmes and her work with learners and patients have influenced our work and our books greatly.

We are particularly grateful to Bob Berrington and Arthur Hibble for providing protected time for us to write a manual for GP facilitators in the East Anglian Region in 1996. This protected time provided a considerable impetus for the writing of this book. We also thank them for their continuing and enthusiastic support of communication skills training in East Anglia.

We are similarly grateful to Annette La Grange and Ian Winchester (Faculty of Education) and Penny Jennett, Al Jones, Henry Mandin, Eldon Smith and Wally Temple (Faculty of Medicine) for the sabbatical they made available to Professor Kurtz in 1996 to work on this book and for their ongoing and substantial administrative support of communication programmes at the University of Calgary.

For their advice, help and encouragement we also sincerely thank Peter Campion, Arthur Clark, Brian Gromoff, David Haslam, Renee Martin, Tony Pearson, Meredith Simon and Sue Weaver.

Introduction

An evidence-based approach

The authors of this book believe passionately in the importance of communication skills in medicine: our overriding objective in writing this book and its companion has been to help improve the standard of doctor–patient communication. But belief and passion are not enough to produce changes in medical education or clinical practice. Without evidence to back our claims that improving doctors' communication skills results in better outcomes for patients and doctors, we cannot expect a relatively new discipline such as communication to make substantial inroads into an already crowded curriculum of learning, whether in undergraduate, residency or continuing medical education.

So our aim for this book is to provide an evidence-based approach to communication skills in medicine. We wish not only to demonstrate how to use communication skills in the medical interview but also to provide the research evidence that validates their importance and documents the potential gains to both doctors and patients alike. There is now comprehensive theoretical and research evidence to guide the choice of communication skills to include in the communication curriculum – we know which skills can actually make a difference to clinical practice. These research findings should now inform the educational process and drive the communication skills curriculum forward (Stewart and Roter 1989). In this book, we provide this evidence to help learners, facilitators and programme directors to understand fully the theoretical and research basis of the subject. This book therefore strives to:

- enhance the communication skills of *students, residents* and *established practitioners of medicine*
- provide *learners, facilitators* and *programme directors* with the research evidence and knowledge to understand and teach this vital subject
- convince *medical educators* of the importance of developing extensive and excellent communication skills programmes within their institutions.

In our companion book *Teaching and Learning Communication Skills in Medicine*, we explore how to actively use the evidence described here in communication skills teaching. We present teaching and learning methods that enable the evidence not only to be used in formal presentations but, more importantly, to be introduced opportunistically to help illuminate and deepen experiential small group or one-to-one learning.

A skills-based approach

In our companion book we identify three areas that communication skills programmes need to address: skills, attitudes and issues. We emphasize the importance of a skills-based approach and how it should be seen as the final common pathway for all communication learning. This book therefore focuses specifically on skills rather than attitudes or issues. We define a curriculum of core communication skills, document how to use these skills in the medical interview and describe the theoretical and research evidence that substantiates their value.

Core skills are fundamental: once they have been mastered, more specific communication issues and challenges such as anger, addiction, breaking bad news or cultural issues are much more readily tackled. Many previously published texts quickly move on to these specific issues after only a brief description of core skills. Our aim is to redress this balance. We wish to provide a secure platform of core skills which will serve as the primary resource for dealing with all communication challenges and upon which issue-specific skills can be superimposed when necessary. The core skills that we describe are the foundation for doctor–patient communication in all circumstances.

A co-ordinated approach to communication skills teaching throughout undergraduate, residency and continuing medical education

We are especially keen to tie together the teaching of communication skills in undergraduate, residency and continuing medical education. In our own work we use the same principles of learning and teach the same core skills in all three settings. We wish to demonstrate the need for a continuing, coherent programme of communication skills teaching that extends throughout all three levels of medical education, the need to both review and reiterate previous learning and the importance of deepening skills and moving on to more complex challenges as learners advance from one level to the next. The curriculum of core skills that we offer provides a common foundation for communication programmes throughout undergraduate, residency and continuing medical education.

A unified approach to communication skills teaching in specialist and family medicine

Some commentators have suggested that it is not possible for a text on communication skills teaching and learning to be appropriate to both general practice and the wide range of settings found in specialist medicine as these different contexts require very different skills. We disagree and feel strongly that these arguments have in the past been responsible for holding back the expansion of communication training. As many of the concepts and research efforts concerning communication skills were initially forged in general practice or psychiatry, it has been easy for other specialists to say that the findings are irrelevant to the special needs of their work and that the lessons from one discipline cannot be transferred to another. The authors have considerable experience in teaching communication across a wide range of specialties and we have observed doctors' and medical students' communication skills in a wide variety of settings. While different contexts may require a subtle shift in emphasis, our overwhelming common experience is that the similarities far outweigh the differences and that the underlying principles and core communication skills remain the same; the barriers between specialties are more in subject matter than in communication skills. In this book we present evidence from a variety of diverse specialist settings which lends support to this approach.

A unified approach to communication skills teaching which crosses cultural and national boundaries

It has also been said that there are such important differences in culture, patient expectations, medical training, clinical management and health care systems between Britain, North America and other countries that it is very difficult to write a book on communication skills that appeals to such a wide audience. Again, we disagree. The authors use the same principles of learning and teach the same basic skills both in England and in Canada. Professor Kurtz, in particular, has observed medical consultations and collaborated on improving medical communication in many countries and cultures and, again, the similarities are far greater than the differences. Strangely, research and theory have not always travelled well between countries and teaching programmes tend not to take account of the progress made elsewhere. The Toronto consensus statement (Simpson *et al.* 1991), multi-authored books such as Stewart and Roter's *Communicating with medical patients* (1989) and international conferences have started to break down these international barriers. We would like to continue the process with this book.

Who are the intended audience for this book?
Learners at all levels of medical education

This book is intended as core material for learners in communication skills programmes, whether at undergraduate, residency or continuing medical education levels. We are keen for learners to read this book to complement their experiential training. We emphasize, however, that reading alone cannot replace experiential learning. As we discuss in our companion book on teaching and learning, cognitive knowledge by itself does not change learners' behaviour in the consultation: experiential methods are required to cement learning from knowledge-based methods into place. However, knowledge does allow learners to understand more fully just what each skill involves, the evidence for each skill leading to improved outcomes in the consultation and the issues behind communication skills training. Intellectual understanding can greatly augment and guide our use of skills and aid our exploration of attitudes.

Facilitators and programme directors

Another major audience for our book are the facilitators and programme directors who wish to teach, plan and develop communication skills training programmes, whether in under-graduate, residency or continuing medical education. As we discuss in our companion book, facilitators and programme directors need help with both the 'what' and the 'how' of com-munication skills teaching. Most medically trained facilitators and programme directors were themselves educated in an era when communication skills were hardly taught at all. Too often it has been assumed that facilitators, through their very practice of medicine, will have gained sufficient knowledge of the specific skills involved in medical communication – the 'what' of communication skills teaching – and that all they need to learn is 'how' to teach this subject. We place equal emphasis on training facilitators and programme directors in both the 'what' and the 'how'. Both are vitally important. Our companion book tackles 'how' to teach, here we help facilitators and programme directors to increase their knowledge of 'what' to teach and to understand the research basis of communication in medicine.

We recognize that facilitators and programme directors are not a uniform group and may come from the following very diverse backgrounds:

- Medical
  - community, hospital or academic-based doctors
  - general practice and family practice physicians
  - psychiatrists
  - specialists
  - nurses
  - allied health professionals
- Non-medical
  - communication specialists
  - psychology or counselling backgrounds.

This diversity has caused some stylistic difficulties. In the book we have often chosen to refer to facilitators as if they are all doctors – we might quote the facilitator as saying to a learner group '*we* all have similar problems with patients' even though our readers, like the three authors of this book, are not all medical practitioners. We use this device because we feel it is sometimes preferable to saying 'what you doctors all do is …'; it is helpful to include our-selves in such descriptions even if we are not all doctors so as to align ourselves with the medical profession rather than seem to be 'doctor-bashing'. Those of us who are not doctors have interactions with our learners that are similar to those doctors have with their patients and the lessons to be learnt are very similar for us all. Hopefully, non-medical facilitators will understand that we are not implying that all facilitators are or should be doctors.

Medical education administrators, funding agencies and medical politicians

It is vital that the importance of communication skills teaching is understood by those in positions of authority and power – deans of medical institutions, administrators of health management organizations (HMOs), hospitals and health authorities, medical societies, royal colleges, medical associations, funding agencies and medical politicians. It is also vital that this audience appreciates the complexity of the communication curriculum and the scholarship that underpins and validates this subject.

How have we addressed style issues in a book intended for both a European and North American market?

A particular problem of this book has been how to write for a diverse audience. So many words and phrases have subtly different meanings that we have had to tread carefully to avoid unnecessary confusion. Throughout the book we have decided to use certain words consistently; we apologize for this shorthand and hope that readers will be able to translate our convention to fit their own context. For instance, we have tried to use:

specialist rather than *consultant*
resident rather than *registrar* or *trainee*
programme director rather than *course organizer*
facilitator rather than *preceptor* or *trainer*
learner rather than *student*
office rather than *surgery*
follow-up visit rather than *review.*

Some areas have proved to be more difficult. We use *medical interview, consultation* and *session* interchangeably. We also use the British *general practice* and North American *family medicine* to mean the same, despite their different meanings in North America.

1

Defining what to teach and learn: an overview of the communication skills curriculum

Introduction

In our companion book, *Teaching and Learning Communication Skills in Medicine,* we presented a detailed rationale for communication skills training which showed that:

- doctor–patient communication is central to clinical practice
  - doctors perform 200 000 consultations in a professional lifetime so it is worth struggling to get it right
  - there are major problems in communication between doctors and patients
  - effective communication is essential to high-quality medicine; it improves patient satisfaction, recall, understanding, adherence and outcomes of care
- communication is a core clinical skill, an essential component of clinical competence
  - knowledge, communication skills, physical examination and problem solving are the four essential components of clinical competence and the very essence of good clinical practice
  - communication skills are not an optional extra; without appropriate communication skills, our knowledge and intellectual efforts are easily wasted
  - communication turns theory into practice; how we communicate is just as important as what we say

- communication skills need to be taught and learned
  - communication is a series of skills that can be both learned and retained; it is not just a personality trait
  - experience alone can be a poor teacher
  - communication needs to be taught with the same rigour as other core skills such as the physical examination
- specific teaching and learning methods are required in communication skills training
  - a skills-based approach is essential to achieve change in learners' behaviour
  - experiential learning methods incorporating observation, feedback and rehearsal are required
  - a problem-based approach to communication skills learning is necessary
  - cognitive and attitudinal learning complement a skills-based approach.

We hope to have convinced our readers not only that teaching and learning communication skills are of the utmost importance but also that appropriate teaching methods can produce effective and long-lasting change in learners' communication skills.

In this book, we develop a theme introduced in our companion volume, i.e. by undertaking communication skills training we can improve our clinical practice (Box 1.1).

Box 1.1   The prize on offer from communication skills training is improved clinical performance

---

- Communication is not just 'being nice' but produces a more effective consultation for both patient and doctor.
- Effective communication improves accuracy, efficiency and supportiveness in the consultation.
- Effective communication significantly improves health outcomes for patients.
- Communication bridges the gap between evidence-based medicine and working with individual patients.

More effective consultations

Throughout this book, we return to the concepts outlined in Box 1.1 and examine how communication skills produce more *effective* consultations for both doctor and patient. We show how communication skills make history taking and problem solving more *accurate* and explore how attention to communication skills helps us to be more *supportive* to patients.

In particular, we stress how the appropriate use of communication skills enables us to be more *efficient* in day-to-day practice. We are not interested in promoting skills that are inappropriate to the time constraints within which we have to practise medicine in the real world. We argue throughout this book that using the communication skills suggested will enhance efficiency and we take pains to provide evidence to validate our assertions.

Improved health outcomes

We will also see how effective communication can significantly improve *health outcomes* for patients. Throughout this book, we relate the use of individual skills to improvements in the following parameters of care: patient satisfaction, adherence, symptom relief and physiological outcome.

To substantiate these claims for improvements in patient care, this book takes an *evidence-based approach* to communication skills that not only describes the skills and demonstrates their use in the medical interview but also provides the research and theoretical evidence that validate their importance and document the potential gains for both doctor and patient alike.

Communication can also improve outcomes for doctors. We will see how the use of appropriate communication skills not only increases patient satisfaction with their doctor but also helps doctors feel less frustrated and more satisfied in their work.

A collaborative partnership

The skills we identify encourage a *patient-centred approach* that promotes a *collaborative partnership* between patient and doctor. This is not because of our own subjective opinion or personal beliefs – we take this approach because the skills that enable this theoretical view of the doctor–patient relationship to be achieved have been shown both in practice and in research to produce better outcomes for patients and doctors.

The concept of a collaborative partnership implies a more equal relationship between patient and doctor and a shift in the balance of power away from medical paternalism towards mutuality. This book explores the communication skills that doctors can employ to enhance their patients' ability to become more involved in the consultation and to take part in a more balanced relationship.

However, there is a further dimension of equal importance which is beyond the scope of this book – what patients can do in the interview to influence communication and their own health care. Far from being passive recipients of changes that doctors adopt, patients have a major part to play in the process of the consultation. How individual patients can participate differently in the consultation, how they can take responsibility themselves to alter the doctor–patient relationship, how they can adopt a more active role in the interview are questions that deserve equal attention and investigation. Although this book touches on research that demonstrates the value of providing patients with skills to enable them to adopt a more active role in the medical interview, here we concentrate on what doctors can do in the interview to facilitate their patients' involvement.

Plan of chapter

The next five chapters follow through the sequence of the medical interview and examine each individual skill in depth; they provide learners and teachers with a detailed understanding of the skills of medical communication. But first, to make the skills easier to understand

and use, we provide an overview of what to teach and learn in the communication skills curriculum. In this chapter we therefore explore the following key questions:

- What are the skills?
  Is it possible to break down such a complex, worthy and important task as the medical interview into its individual components? Can we identify and define the individual skills that together constitute medical communication and that we wish to include in the communication curriculum?
- How do the skills fit together?
  Can we present the skills within an overall conceptual framework that enables learners and teachers to make sense of the skills themselves and how they relate to the consultation as a whole?
- Is there evidence that these skills make a difference in doctor–patient communication?
  What is the theoretical and research basis that justifies the inclusion of the skills in our communication programmes? Is there good evidence for the efficacy of these skills or is it all subjective opinion?

Defining the broad types of communication skills

In our companion volume, we demonstrated that three broad types of skills need to be included in communication skills training:

1 **Content skills.** What doctors communicate – the substance of their questions and responses; the information they gather and give; the treatments they discuss
2 **Process skills.** How they do it – the ways they communicate with patients; how they go about discovering the history or providing information; the verbal and non-verbal skills they use; how they develop the relationship with the patient; the way they organize and structure communication
3 **Perceptual skills.** What they are thinking and feeling – their internal decision making, clinical reasoning and problem solving; their awareness of feelings and thoughts about the patient, the illness and other issues that may be concerning them; awareness of their own self-concept and confidence, of their own biases, attitudes, intentions and distractions.

Content, process and perceptual skills are inextricably linked and need to be considered in unison in communication teaching. This book focuses deliberately on process skills and on how they influence and are influenced by perceptual skills and, to a lesser degree, content skills. Although content skills such as the questions that constitute the family history and the functional enquiry are vitally important, they are well described in many traditional textbooks and we devote little space to them here. It is the process skills that are less well described. Because these are the skills that most require definition and exploration, it is process skills and their interactions with perceptual skills that we examine in depth in this book.

An overall curriculum of skills: the *Calgary–Cambridge observation guide*

We present our overview of what to teach and learn in the form of the *Calgary–Cambridge observation guide*, the centrepiece of our whole approach to communication skills teaching and a major feature of both books. The guide provides a concise and accessible summary of the communication skills curriculum. It both establishes the structure that we follow throughout this book and serves as an *aide-mémoire* of the individual skills that we discuss.

We stress that the guide does not just summarize the 'what' of the communication curriculum; it is also an important part of the 'how' of communication skills teaching and learning. In our companion book, we provide a more detailed presentation of how to use the guide as a teaching and learning tool. Here, we repeat the rationale for the guide's derivation and approach.

The *Calgary–Cambridge observation guide* (Kurtz and Silverman 1996) addresses the four main issues which influence what to teach and learn in skills-based communication programmes:

1 **structure:** how do we organize communication skills?
2 **skills:** what are the skills that we are trying to promote?
3 **validity:** what evidence is there that these skills make a difference in doctor–patient communication?
4 **breadth:** what is the scope of the communication curriculum?

The guide was developed as a teaching tool to provide answers to the above questions in an accessible and practical format that would be helpful to learners and facilitators alike. The guide has two broad aims. Firstly, to help facilitators and students conceptualize and structure their teaching and learning. Secondly, to assist communication programme directors, whether working in undergraduate, residency or continuing medical education, in their efforts to establish training programmes for both learners and facilitators.

In three pages, the guide:

- proposes a framework for organizing the skills of medical communication that corresponds directly to the way we structure the consultation and therefore aids teaching, learning and medical practice
- delineates and describes the individual skills that make up the curriculum of medical communication skills training programmes
- summarizes and makes accessible the literature regarding each area of value in communication skills teaching
- forms the foundation of a comprehensive curriculum (Riccardi and Kurtz 1983; Kurtz 1989), providing learners, facilitators and programme directors alike with a clear idea of the curriculum's learning objectives
- provides a concise summary of the skills for both facilitators and learners which they can use on an everyday basis during teaching sessions as an accessible *aide-mémoire* and a way to structure observation, feedback and self-evaluation
- provides a common language for labelling and referring to specific behaviours

- provides a sound basis for the content of facilitator training programmes, creating coherence and consistency in the teaching of the large number of facilitators required in a communication programme
- provides a common foundation for communication programmes at all levels of training – undergraduate, residency and continuing medical education – by specifying a comprehensive set of core patient–doctor communication skills, equally valid and applicable in all three contexts.

Although in the past many people have clarified what to teach and numerous guides and check-lists have been available, including our own previous versions (Stillman *et al.* 1976; Cassata 1978; Sanson-Fisher 1981; Riccardi and Kurtz 1983; Cohen-Cole 1991; van Thiel *et al.* 1991; Novack *et al.* 1992), the *Calgary–Cambridge observation guide* makes significant advances by:

- taking into account the current moves to a more patient-centred and collaborative approach
- referencing the list of skills in line with current research and theory
- increasing the emphasis on the extremely important area of explanation and planning (Carroll and Monroe 1979; Riccardi and Kurtz 1983; Maguire *et al.* 1986; Tuckett *et al.* 1985; Sanson-Fisher *et al.* 1991).

We are particularly indebted to Dr Rob Sanson-Fisher (Australia) for his contributions to the structure of parts of the guide and to Drs Vincent Riccardi (USA) and Catherine Heaton (Canada). Earlier editions of the guide have been used successfully for the last 20 years as a central feature of teaching in the undergraduate communication curriculum at the University of Calgary Faculty of Medicine in Canada (Riccardi and Kurtz 1983; Kurtz 1989). More recently, the guide has also been adapted for wider use to include family medicine, internal medicine and other residents as well as practising physicians. It has been introduced into the teaching of British general practice residents and their facilitators in the East Anglian region and refined through a process of experimentation in workshops with practising physicians and facilitators. It is equally suited to both small group and one-to-one teaching.

The structure of the *Calgary–Cambridge observation guide*

The guide uses a simple five-point plan within which the individual skills are structured. This plan is based on the five basic tasks that physicians and patients routinely attempt to accomplish in everyday clinical practice. Physicians and patients tend to carry out these tasks roughly in sequence, with the exception of relationship building, a task which is performed continuously throughout the interview. The tasks therefore make intuitive sense and provide a logical, organizational schema for both physician–patient interactions and communication skills education. This structure was first proposed by Riccardi and Kurtz in 1983 and is similar to that adopted by Cohen-Cole in 1991.

THE TASKS

1 **Initiating the session**
2 **Gathering information**
3 **Building the relationship**
4 **Explanation and planning**
5 **Closing the session**

An expanded framework of skills sets then provides further details of the steps to be achieved within each consultation.

THE EXPANDED FRAMEWORK

1 **Initiating the session:**
   - establishing initial rapport
   - identifying the reason(s) for the consultation
2 **Gathering information:**
   - exploration of problems
   - understanding the patient's perspective
   - providing structure to the consultation
3 **Building the relationship:**
   - developing rapport
   - involving the patient
4 **Explanation and planning:**
   - providing the correct amount and type of information
   - aiding accurate recall and understanding
   - achieving a shared understanding: incorporating the patient's perspective
   - planning: shared decision making
   - options in explanation and planning
     - if discussing opinion and significance of problems
     - if negotiating mutual plan of action
     - if discussing investigations and procedures
5 **Closing the session**

The skills of the *Calgary–Cambridge observation guide*

The guide then lists the *individual* skills within this framework:

Initiating the session

Establishing initial rapport
1 Greets patient and obtains patient's name
2 Introduces self and clarifies role
3 Demonstrates interest and respect, attends to patient's physical comfort

Identifying the reason(s) for the consultation
4 The opening question: identifies the problems or issues that the patient wishes to address (e.g. 'What would you like to discuss today?')
5 Listening to the patient's opening statement: listens attentively, without interrupting or directing patient's response
6 Screening: checks and confirms list of problems (e.g. 'So that's headaches and tiredness. Is there anything else you'd like to discuss today?')
7 Agenda setting: negotiates agenda, taking both patient's and physician's needs into account

Gathering information

Exploration of problems
8 Patient's narrative: encourages patient to tell the story of the problem(s), from when first started to the present, in own words (clarifying reason for presenting now)
9 Question style: uses open and closed questioning techniques, appropriately moving from open to closed
10 Listening: listens attentively, allowing patient to complete statements without interruption and leaving space for patient to think before answering or go on after pausing
11 Facilitative response: facilitates patient's responses verbally and non-verbally (e.g. use of encouragement, silence, repetition, paraphrasing, interpretation)
12 Clarification: checks out statements which are vague or need amplification (e.g. 'Could you explain what you mean by light-headed?')
13 Internal summary: periodically summarizes to verify own understanding of what the patient has said; invites patient to correct interpretation or provide further information
14 Language: uses concise, easily understood questions and comments; avoids or adequately explains jargon

Understanding the patient's perspective
15 Ideas and concerns: determines and acknowledges patient's ideas (i.e. beliefs re cause) and concerns (i.e. worries) regarding each problem
16 Effects: determines how each problem affects the patient's life
17 Expectations: determines patient's goals, what help the patient had expected for each problem
18 Feelings and thoughts: encourages expression of the patient's feelings and thoughts
19 Cues: picks up verbal and non-verbal cues (body language, speech, facial expression, affect); checks out and acknowledges as appropriate

Providing structure to the consultation

20 Internal summary: summarizes at the end of a specific line of inquiry to confirm understanding before moving on to the next section

21 Signposting: progresses from one section to another using transitional statements; includes rationale for next section

22 Sequencing: structures interview in logical sequence

23 Timing: attends to timing and keeping interview on task

Building the relationship

Developing rapport

24 Non-verbal behaviour: demonstrates appropriate non-verbal behaviour (e.g. eye contact, posture and position, movement, facial expression, use of voice)

25 Use of notes: if reads, writes notes or uses computer, does in a manner that does not interfere with dialogue or rapport

26 Acceptance: acknowledges patient's views and feelings; accepts legitimacy; is not judgemental

27 Empathy and support: expresses concern, understanding, willingness to help; acknowledges coping efforts and appropriate self-care

28 Sensitivity: deals sensitively with embarrassing and disturbing topics and physical pain, including when associated with physical examination

Involving the patient

29 Sharing of thoughts: shares thinking with patient as appropriate to encourage patient's involvement, enhance understanding (e.g. 'What I'm thinking now is …')

30 Provides rationale: explains rationale for questions or parts of physical examination that could appear to be non-sequiturs

31 Examination: during physical examination, explains process, asks permission

Explanation and planning

Providing the correct amount and type of information

Aims: to give comprehensive and appropriate information
        to assess each individual patient's information needs
        to neither restrict nor overload

32 Chunks and checks: gives information in assimilable chunks, checks for understanding, uses patient's response as a guide to how to proceed

33 Assesses patient's starting point: asks for patient's prior knowledge early on when giving information; discovers extent of patient's wish for information

34 Asks patients what other information would be helpful (e.g. aetiology, prognosis)

35 Gives explanation at appropriate times: avoids giving advice, information or reassurance prematurely

Aiding accurate recall and understanding

Aims: to make information easier for the patient to remember and understand

36 Organizes explanation: divides into discrete sections; develops a logical sequence

37 Uses explicit categorization or signposting (e.g. 'There are three important things that I would like to discuss. First ...'; 'Now, shall we move on to ...')
38 Uses repetition and summarizing: to reinforce information
39 Language: uses concise, easily understood statements; avoids or explains jargon
40 Uses visual methods of conveying information: diagrams, models, written information and instructions
41 Checks patient's understanding of information given (or plans made), e.g. by asking patient to restate in own words; clarifies as necessary

Achieving a shared understanding: incorporating the patient's perspective
Aims: to provide explanations and plans that relate to the patient's perspective of the problem
        to discover the patient's thoughts and feelings about the information given
        to encourage an interaction rather than one-way transmission

42 Relates explanations to patient's illness framework: to previously elicited ideas, concerns and expectations
43 Provides opportunities and encourages patient to contribute: to ask questions, seek clarification or express doubts; responds appropriately
44 Picks up verbal and non-verbal cues, e.g. patient's need to contribute information or ask questions; information overload; distress
45 Elicits patient's beliefs, reactions and feelings re information given, terms used; acknowledges and addresses where necessary

Planning: shared decision making
Aims: to allow patients to understand the decision-making process
        to involve patients in decision making to the level they wish
        to increase patients' commitment to plans made

46 Shares own thoughts: ideas, thought processes and dilemmas as appropriate
47 Involves patient by making suggestions rather than directives
48 Encourages patient to contribute their thoughts: ideas, suggestions and preferences
49 Negotiates a mutually acceptable plan
50 Offers choices: encourages patient to make choices and decisions to the level that they wish
51 Checks with patient: if plan acceptable; if concerns have been addressed

Closing the session

52 End summary: summarizes session briefly and clarifies plan of care
53 Contracting: contracts with patient re next steps for patient and physician
54 Safety netting: explains possible unexpected outcomes; what to do if plan is not working; when and how to seek help
55 Final checking: checks that patient agrees and is comfortable with plan and asks if any corrections, questions or other items to discuss

Options in explanation and planning

If discussing opinion and significance of problems
56 Offers opinion of what is going on and names if possible
57 Reveals rationale for opinion

58 Explains causation, seriousness, expected outcome, short and long-term consequences

59 Elicits patient's beliefs, reactions and concerns, e.g. if opinion matches patient's thoughts, acceptability, feelings

If negotiating mutual plan of action

60 Discusses options, e.g. no action; investigation; medication or surgery; non-drug treatments [physiotherapy, walking aids, fluids, counselling]; preventative measures

61 Provides information on action or treatment offered, e.g. name; steps involved; how it works; benefits and advantages; possible side-effects

62 Obtains patient's view of need for action, perceived benefits, barriers, motivation

63 Accepts patient's views; advocates alternative viewpoint as necessary

64 Elicits patient's reactions and concerns about plans and treatments, including acceptability

65 Takes patient's lifestyle, beliefs, cultural background and abilities into consideration

66 Encourages patient to be involved in implementing plans, to take responsibility and be self-reliant

67 Asks about patient support systems; discusses other support available

If discussing investigations and procedures

68 Provides clear information on procedures, including what patient might experience and how patient will be informed of results

69 Relates procedures to treatment plan: value and purpose

70 Encourages questions about, and discussion of, potential anxieties or negative outcomes

The need for a structure

An important element of the curriculum that we have described above is the provision of a clear, overall structure within which the individual communication skills are organized. We refer to this conceptual framework repeatedly throughout the book. Why do we place such importance on defining such an overt structure?

An understanding of structure has benefits for practitioners, learners and facilitators alike:

- **For practitioners**, an awareness of structure prevents the consultation from wandering aimlessly and important points from being missed. For instance, without recognizing that the gathering information phase of the interview involves developing an understanding of the patient's individual reaction to their illness as well as the biomedical aspects of their disease, the doctor may enter the explanation and planning phase of the interview prematurely and fail to address the patient's real concerns. Of course, an awareness of structure in the consultation has to be combined with flexibility: consultations do not have a fixed path that can be dictated by the doctor without reference to the patient. But without structure, it is all too easy for communication to be unsystematic and unproductive.
- **For learners at all levels**, a list of the individual communication skills alone is not sufficient. Learners also need an overall conceptual framework to help organize the skills into a memorable and useful whole. In our companion book, we see the importance of experiential methods in producing change in learners' communication skills. Experiential teaching is, however, intrinsically random and opportunistic, and the feedback and suggestions made in experiential work can be difficult to pull together. Providing a structure into which skills can be placed as they arise helps learners to order the skills that they discover opportunistically in experiential work and to see how the individual pieces fit together into the consultation as a whole.
- **Facilitators** may also lack a clear idea of how to pull together the individual skills that they recognize as important learning areas. The numerous skills of the medical interview often appear to be a disorganized bag of tricks without any overall framework. Facilitators can find it difficult to link the different skills together in their teaching. A clear and overt structure can help overcome this problem. Structure has the added advantage of enabling facilitators to take an outcome-based approach in their communication skills teaching. Structure establishes an overview, enabling facilitators to ask two central questions of learners: 'Where are you in the interview?' and 'What are you and the patient trying to achieve?'. Having established a direction, the individual skills then help with the next question, 'How might you get there?'.

Choosing the skills to include in the communication curriculum

We are well aware that the extensive list of skills included in the guide can initially be rather daunting to new learners and facilitators. We can almost hear the reader saying 'You must be joking. Seventy skills to learn, assimilate and master: that's impossible!'. Does it really need to be that complicated? Couldn't we reduce the numbers or amalgamate a few items? Is it really necessary to try to incorporate all these skills into each consultation?

Our unapologetic answer to this is that the medical interview is indeed very complex and cannot be summed up in a few broad generalizations. Communication is a series of learned skills and it is both possible and essential to break the consultation down into these individual skills if we wish to identify, practise and assimilate new behaviours into our practice of medicine. All of the skills listed in the guide can be of great value to the process and outcome of the interview; all, as we will see below, have been validated by theory or research and all will repay our learners' attention.

However, we are not suggesting that every skill needs to be employed on every occasion. For instance, although most of the skills in the gathering information phase of the interview are appropriate to every consultation, the use of many of the skills in the explanation and planning phase needs to be tailored to the individual circumstances of the interview – they will not be used in every consultation. However, familiarity with all of the skills will undoubtedly be of benefit. At the very least, they can then be used intentionally and deliberately whenever the going gets tough and danger looms!

But what is the basis for the inclusion of each of the 70 listed skills in the Calgary–Cambridge curriculum? Are we able to validate the importance of each of these skills in any way or is it purely subjective opinion? Where does the justification for these particular skills come from?

The research and theoretical bases that validate the inclusion of each individual skill

It is no longer appropriate to consider communication skills teaching as simply raising awareness of the importance of communication in the consultation. Nor is it just a matter of sharing various approaches, increasing the range of possibilities available or treating all suggestions as equally valid. Certain skills and methods have now been shown to make a substantial difference to doctor–patient communication and to ensuing health outcomes.

We are fortunate that over the last 25 years an extensive canon of theoretical and research evidence has accumulated which enables us to define the skills that enhance communication between patient and physician. Research clearly demonstrates how the use of individual skills can lead to improvements in patient satisfaction, adherence, symptom relief and physiological outcome. We can now promote these skills as worth teaching and encouraging within a communication programme. We are able to confidently answer the question 'Where's the validity?' and effectively counter the suggestion that communication skills are purely subjective.

The curriculum of skills is not and should not be static: research will continue to accumulate to challenge our preconceptions and move the goalposts of communication skills teaching. For instance, in recent years research findings have enabled the curriculum to shift in two important directions. Firstly, there has been increasing emphasis on the important but often previously neglected field of explanation and planning (information giving). Secondly, there has been a move towards a more patient-centred and collaborative approach.

In this chapter, we have simply delineated a curriculum for communication skills training programmes by listing and defining each skill. In the remaining chapters of the book, we will examine the research and theoretical evidence that validate each individual skill.

The underlying principles of communication that have helped guide us in choosing the skills

Along with the research evidence, three immediate *goals* (Box 1.2) and five *principles* of communication (Box 1.3) also helped in the choice of skills to include in the guide. Together, they combine to provide a simple and coherent theoretical foundation for the guide and for the development of communication curricula in general. We will refer to these goals and principles throughout the remaining chapters of the book to illustrate the importance of individual skills.

Box 1.2   Goals of medical communication

The three immediate goals that physicians attempt to achieve whenever they talk to patients are:

1 accuracy
2 efficiency
3 supportiveness.

Effective communication provides the means of accomplishing these goals (Riccardi and Kurtz 1983).

Skills and individuality

Each skill listed in the guide is only a clue to learners and facilitators that this is an area where specific behaviours and phrases need to be developed. The list by itself is not enough; each learner has to discover his own way to put each skill into practice. While the guide identifies the skills that have been shown to be of value in doctor–patient communication, it does not attempt to specify exact or recommended ways of accomplishing them. The task of communication skills teaching is to give participants the opportunity to try out phrases and behaviours that fit their own individual personalities and to extend the repertoire of skills with which each participant is comfortable.

Structure: Where am I in the consultation and what do I want to achieve?
Specific skills: How do I get there?
Phrasing or behaviour: How can I incorporate these skills into my own style and personality?

Going beyond specific skills into individuality is the real challenge of experiential learning. We cannot and should not be prescriptive about the best way to proceed in any circumstance. We must recognize that there are enormous variables that influence what is best for you as an individual in a given situation. But we must also recognize that we can now advocate certain skills that are likely to be more effective than others.

Box 1.3   Principles that characterize effective communication

---

The following five principles, applicable to any setting, help us to understand what constitutes effective communication (Kurtz 1989).

Effective communication:

1 *ensures an interaction rather than a direct transmission process.* If communication is viewed as a direct transmission process, the senders of messages can assume that their responsibilities as communicators are fulfilled once they have formulated and sent a message. However, if communication is viewed as an interactive process, the interaction is complete only if the sender receives feedback about how the message is interpreted, whether it is understood and what impact it has on the receiver. Just imparting information or just listening is not enough: giving and receiving feedback about the impact of the message becomes crucial. The emphasis moves to the interdependence of sender and receiver, and the contributions and initiatives of each become more equal in importance (Dance and Larson 1972). The aim of communication becomes the establishment of mutually understood common ground (Baker 1955).

2 *reduces unnecessary uncertainty.* It is important to consider all possible causes of uncertainty in the medical interview. Unresolved uncertainties in any area can lead to lack of concentration or anxiety which in turn can block effective communication. For example, patients may be uncertain about what to expect during a given interview, about the significance of a line of questioning, about the role of a particular member of the health care team, or about the attitudes, intentions or trustworthiness of the interviewer. Reducing uncertainty about diagnosis or expected outcomes of care is obviously important although living with some uncertainty is often a necessity in medical situations. However, even then, openly discussing areas where knowledge is lacking or no one is certain of the best choice can help reduce uncertainty by establishing mutually understood common ground.

3 *requires planning and thinking in terms of outcomes.* The best way to determine effectiveness is to think in terms of outcomes and consequences. If I am angry and the outcome I seek is to vent emotion, I proceed in one direction. However, if the outcome I want is to resolve any problem or misunderstanding that may have caused my anger, I must proceed in a different way to be effective.

4 *demonstrates dynamism.* What is appropriate for one situation is inappropriate for another – different individuals' needs and contexts change continually. What the patient understood so clearly yesterday seems beyond comprehension today. Just as one area of understanding seems to be nearing completion, another avenue opens up. Dynamism underscores the need not only for flexibility but also for responsiveness and involvement.

5 *follows the helical model.* The helical model of communication (Dance 1967) has two implications. Firstly, what I say influences what you say in spiral fashion so that our communication gradually evolves as we interact. Secondly, reiteration and repetition, coming back around the spiral of communication at a slightly different level each time, are essential for effective communication.

It is the repeated trying-out of alternatives in rehearsal, role playing with other learners or practising with simulated or real patients that allows us to reconcile the two concepts of skills and individuality. The list of skills is in itself only a start. To learn how to use each skill requires practice and further feedback, and through this process of repeated practice, feedback and rehearsal, each learner stamps his own individuality on the communication process.

Issue-specific skills

The skills collated in the guide provide the foundations for effective doctor–patient communication in many different medical contexts. However, the list is not all-encompassing: there are circumstances in which additional issue-specific skills are also required, such as breaking bad news, bereavement, revealing hidden depression, gender and cultural issues, prevention and motivation (Gask *et al*. 1988; Maguire and Faulkner 1988; Sanson-Fisher *et al*. 1991; Chugh *et al*. 1993). These issues clearly deserve special attention in our teaching and we will explore them further in Chapter 7. However, we would like to stress that the skills delineated in the guide are the *core* communication skills required in all these circumstances, providing a secure platform on which specific communication issues and challenges can be superimposed.

Summary

In this chapter we have defined an overall curriculum of physician–patient communication skills. We now explore these skills in more detail. What is the rationale for using each skill in the consultation? How is each skill used? What is the research and theoretical evidence that validate each individual skill? The next five chapters examine these issues in depth. The book is organized to follow the structure of the *Calgary–Cambridge observation guide*, each of the five chapters describing the skills that pertain to a section of the guide. We start by looking at the skills required for beginning the consultation.

2

Initiating the session

Introduction

The beginning of the interview is a particularly rich area to explore in communication skills teaching. In these opening minutes we make our first impressions, begin to establish rapport, attempt to identify the problems that the patient wishes to discuss and start to plan a course for the interview. The scene is set for the rest of the consultation. Yet we know from research that many problems in communication occur in this initial phase of the interview. As we shall see, physicians frequently even fail to discover the most important reason for the patient's attendance!

Doctors tend to underestimate the potential difficulties and opportunities of these brief first minutes. In almost every teaching course that we have run, the participants' own agenda at the start of the course emphasizes problems in ending the consultation and in keeping to time. But so often it becomes apparent as the course proceeds that it is the beginning rather than the end of the interview that is the root cause of many of their perceived difficulties.

Consultations in medicine occur in widely differing contexts, from new to review appointments, from hospital to general practice, from the consulting room to the bedside, from the hospice to the home. Although at first sight there are many differences between the beginnings of interviews in these very diverse settings, the overall objectives and individual skills required are remarkably consistent. The problems that both doctors and patients face in the initial stages of an interview are very similar wherever they meet.

The specific communication skills that doctors choose to demonstrate at the beginning of the consultation are not merely social niceties; they have an important impact on the accuracy and efficiency of the interview and on the nature of the doctor–patient relationship. We therefore set apart initiation as a separate task and devote a whole chapter to discussing what will take at most only a few minutes to achieve in real time.

Problems in communication

One of the aims at the beginning of any consultation is to identify what the patient wishes to discuss. Here the research evidence from a series of studies in primary care reveals some particularly salutary lessons:

- Stewart *et al.* (1979) showed that 54% of patients' complaints and 45% of their concerns were not elicited
- Starfield *et al.* (1981) recorded that in 50% of visits, the patient and the doctor did not agree on the nature of the main presenting problem
- Burack and Carpenter (1983) found that patients and doctors agreed on the chief complaint in only 76% of somatic problems and in only 6% of psychosocial problems
- Beckman and Frankel (1984) showed that doctors frequently interrupted patients so soon after they began their opening statement – after a mean time of only 18 seconds! – that they failed to disclose other equally significant concerns
- Byrne and Long (1976) found that interviews were particularly likely to become dysfunctional if there were shortcomings in the part of the consultation relating to 'discovering the reason for the patient's attendance'.

Clearly, there is little point in being an excellent diagnostician or possessing great factual knowledge if you are not dealing with the patient's most important problem!

Objectives

We begin our exploration of the initiation phase of the interview by looking at objectives, at what we are hoping to achieve. One of the principles of effective communication that we outlined in Chapter 1 is that *communication requires planning and thinking in terms of outcomes.* It is therefore important in communication to consider our objectives. Objectives make us think about 'Where do we want to get to?'; work on individual skills provides strategies for 'How do we get there?'.
  Objectives include:

- establishing a supportive environment and initial rapport
- developing an awareness of the patient's emotional state
- identifying as far as possible *all* the problems or issues that the patient has come to discuss
- establishing with the patient a mutually agreed agenda or plan for the consultation
- developing a partnership with the patient, enabling the patient to become part of a collaborative process.

These objectives encompass many of the tasks and checkpoints mentioned in other well-known guides to the consultation:

Byrne and Long (1976)   Phase 1: the doctor establishes a relationship with the patient
                          Phase 2: the doctor either attempts to discover or actually discovers the reason for the patient's attendance

Pendleton *et al.* (1984)   To define the reason for the patient's attendance; to establish or maintain a relationship with the patient

Neighbour (1987)   Connecting: establishing rapport with the patient; summarizing: 'Have I sufficiently understood why the patient has come to see me?'

Cohen-Cole (1991)   Gathering data to understand the patient's problem(s); developing rapport and responding to the patient's emotions

Keller and Carroll (1994)   Engaging the patient.

Skills

Having established the objectives of the initiation phase, we can turn our attention to the skills which help us to achieve these goals. The following list of skills is adapted from the *Calgary–Cambridge observation guide* (see Chapter 1). Here we have combined the skills listed in the 'Initiating the session' section of the guide with appropriate items from 'Building the relationship' (which has relevance throughout the consultation).

Box 2.1   Skills for initiating the session

Preparation

- Puts aside last task; attends to self-comfort
- Focuses attention and prepares for the next consultation

Establishing initial rapport

- Greets patient and obtains patient's name
- Introduces self and clarifies role
- Demonstrates interest and respect; attends to patient's physical comfort

Identifying the reason(s) for the consultation

- The opening question: identifies the problems or issues that the patient wishes to address (e.g. 'What would you like to discuss today?')
- Listening to the patient's opening statement: listens attentively without interrupting or directing patient's response
- Screening: checks and confirms list of problems or issues that the patient wishes to cover (e.g. 'So that's headaches and tiredness. Is there anything else you would like to discuss today?')
- Agenda setting: negotiates agenda and format of interview, taking both patient's and physician's needs into account

'What' to teach and learn about the initiation – the evidence for the skills

PREPARATION

As we have seen in Chapter 1, *unresolved uncertainties and anxieties can lead to lack of concentration which in turn can block effective communication.* In clinical practice, it is easy for your mind to still be on the last patient or telephone call, the growing queue of patients still to be seen or your own personal needs. You may find yourself still calling up records on the computer or completing the records as you greet the next patient. These thoughts, feelings and actions can so easily get in the way of providing full concentration at the beginning of the consultation. The alternative is to prepare yourself so that you can give your full attention to the patient and are not distracted by other issues at this critical moment. Although this may be just one of many routine consultations of the day for the doctor, for the patient it may be a far more important and significant occasion. The patient is usually entirely focused on the interview to come; it is clearly helpful if the doctor reciprocates with his full concentration.

Suggestions for preparation and achieving full concentration include:

- **putting aside the last task** – making sure that the last consultation will not impinge on the next, making arrangements to return to unresolved issues later
- **attending to your personal needs and comfort** – ensuring that hunger, heat or sleepiness do not disturb your concentration in the next interview
- **shifting focus to the consultation at hand** – preparing as necessary by reading the notes, searching for results or thinking about the patient's history
- **concluding these activities before greeting the patient** – being free to concentrate in as relaxed and focused a way as possible.

This kind of preparation and focus goes deeper than common courtesy and respect. A study looking at family physicians' perceptions of the causes of their self-admitted clinical errors (Ely *et al.* 1995) showed that hurrying and distraction were among the most common causes to which physicians attributed their mistakes.

ESTABLISHING INITIAL RAPPORT

There has been little research into the value of greetings in the medical setting – presumably as it seems so obvious – but the following elements deserve consideration:

- greeting the patient
- introducing yourself
- clarifying your role
- obtaining the patient's name
- demonstrating interest and respect, attending to patient's physical comfort.

Introductions are a fascinating insight into doctors' practice, particularly as they so often seem to be completely omitted! Patients frequently complain that the doctor did not introduce himself, that they were not sure who they were seeing or what his role was within the team.

Greeting the patient and introducing yourself

If you have not met the patient before, it is relatively easy to welcome and introduce yourself using a combination of non-verbal approaches such as handshake, eye contact and smile plus a suitable verbal greeting:

'Hello, I'm Dr Jones. Do come and sit down.'

Doctors often know their patients well and therefore do not need to introduce themselves to every patient. But they sometimes assume that patients know who they are without any evidence that this is so and inappropriately omit a verbal introduction. They assume that if they have seen a patient before, she will remember who they are and therefore there will be no need to introduce themselves again. They may also feel uncomfortable about introducing themselves to patients who they may have met before but cannot now remember. We need to develop ways of overcoming such problems:

'Hello, please come and sit down. Am I right in thinking we haven't met before? My name is Dr Jones.'

Clarifying your role

For the patient, the uncertainty of not knowing who the doctor is or how she fits into their care can be very unsettling. Yet in a study of 50 medical students, Maguire and Rutter (1976) reported that 80% failed to introduce themselves adequately and to explain their intentions. Would it not be helpful for a student to explain her position within the team, the length of time that she has for interviewing the patient, what she will do with the information obtained and how she will relate this information to the doctor in charge of the patient? Would it not be best to state from the outset that the interview is for the student's rather than the patient's prime benefit if that is the case or conversely if this is the only opportunity the patient will have to give their story and ask questions?

'Hello, my name is Catherine Singh. I'm a student doctor working with Dr Ko. I'm learning how to interview patients. I believe Dr Ko suggested to you that I might spend 15 minutes talking to you before he joins us and tries to help you with your problem. Would that still be all right?'

It might be argued that this is superfluous for experienced doctors, especially in some settings such as family practice where both patient and doctor understand the nature of the consultation and the cultural rules of the encounter. But consider the situation in teaching hospitals, health maintenance organizations, interdisciplinary teams and emergency departments. Where many different clinicians may relate to each individual patient, doctors can prevent confusion by carefully explaining their role and the nature of the interview rather than letting things go unsaid and be ripe for possible misinterpretation.

'Hello, I'm Dr Ko. Can I sit here? I'm one of the specialist surgeons attached to the hospital. Your family doctor, Dr Jones, has asked me to see you.'

Obtaining the patient's name

In circumstances where you know the patient well, this is clearly an unnecessary step. But whenever there is a possibility of confusion, it is always advisable to check that you have the correct name and pronunciation and that the patient's name matches that on the chart. Avoid making assumptions about marital status or preferred form of address:

'Hello, I'm Dr Jones. I'm one of the four partners who make up this family practice. Please sit down. Can I just check – is it Mrs Mary French? [pause] I don't think we've met before; what do you prefer that I call you?'

Demonstrating interest and respect, attending to the patient's physical comfort

We cannot emphasize enough the importance of taking steps to build the relationship from the very beginning of the interview. Demonstrating interest, concern and respect for the patient through appropriate verbal and non-verbal behaviour are so important in laying the groundwork for a productive and collaborative relationship.

The doctor's behaviour and demeanour here are vital in enabling the patient to feel welcomed, valued and respected. Taking steps to establish trust and develop the relationship early on will set the scene for efficient and accurate information exchange as the interview unfolds. Because we need to pay attention to this vital area throughout the whole interview and not just at the beginning, we devote all of Chapter 4 to 'Building the relationship'. There we explore the research evidence for the importance of rapport building skills and non-verbal communication in detail.

Virtually everything that we discuss about initiating the interview in this chapter contributes to relationship building by encouraging the patient's contributions and promoting a collaborative approach. We would like to comment further on one particularly important item: attending to the patient's physical comfort.

Environmental factors affect physical and psychological comfort. They influence our position, posture and eye contact, our perception and attitudes and our ability to attend. Are room temperatures set so patients waiting in dressing gowns are comfortable? Is lighting neither glaring nor too dim? Are patient and doctor positioned so that neither must look into the glare of uncurtained windows? In waiting areas are diversions available, such as written materials, aquariums or patient education materials?

Unless problems such as pain, nausea and injury dictate otherwise, most of us are more comfortable talking while sitting in a chair rather than lying down or dangling our legs over the side of an examining table. All the better if the doctor is also seated as this puts both participants on a more equal footing, makes unobtrusive note-taking easier and gives the impression that the doctor is willing to take the time that is needed to give full attention to the patient.

Placing furniture so that doctor and patient can sit at a knee-to-knee angle rather than side by side or directly across from each other is helpful. Positioning communicators on opposite sides of a desk has been found to have an intimidating, competitive or barrier effect (Sommer 1971). People want easy eye contact but not so direct that they cannot readily 'escape'.

As much as possible, talk with patients while they are fully dressed. If sensitive or private matters are discussed, close doors, draw curtains between beds or, if no privacy is possible, at least reassure the patient and be aware that environment-induced uneasiness may inhibit or distract the patient to the point of giving inaccurate or incomplete information. Finally, keep in mind that all these aspects of environment are as likely to influence the doctor as the patient.

IDENTIFYING THE REASON(S) FOR THE CONSULTATION

Having exchanged introductions and established initial rapport, the next step is to determine what issues the patient wishes to discuss. What is their agenda for the interview? Why have they come today? In the context of seeing patients in hospital or at home, doctors need to clarify the problems that the patient wishes to address as well as explaining their own reasons for coming to see the patient.

Perhaps this all seems so obvious as to be hardly worth mentioning. But in fact it is more complicated than we might think. Remember the evidence provided at the beginning of this chapter which showed how often doctors fail to detect problems or issues patients wish to discuss and how frequently doctors and patients disagree after the interview about the nature of the main presenting problem. Clearly, there are problems here that need to be addressed. In fact, the doctor's behaviour and approach during the initiation phase can have profound effects on the rest of the consultation, causing differences not only in the structure and timing of what occurs in the consultation but indeed in the very problems that are discussed.

It is most interesting to compare the evidence from research with some of the common assumptions that doctors make at the beginning of the interview:

- several investigators have shown that patients often have more than one concern to discuss: in a variety of settings, including primary care, paediatrics and internal medicine, the mean number of concerns ranged from 1.2 to 3.9 in both new and return visits (Starfield *et al.* 1981; Good and Good 1982; Wasserman *et al.* 1984; Greenfield *et al.* 1985). These studies warn of the danger of premature and limited hypothesis testing before a wider spectrum of concerns has been identified
- in a study of internal medicine residents and physicians in primary care, Beckman and Frankel (1984) have shown that:
  - the serial order in which patients present their problems is not related to their clinical importance: the first concern presented is no more likely than the second or third to be the most important as judged by either the patient or the doctor
  - doctors very often assume erroneously that the first complaint mentioned is the only one that the patient has brought
  - in follow-up visits, doctors often assume that the consultation is a direct continuation of the last interview and omit the opening solicitation entirely, proceeding directly to questions about concerns elicited in previous visits.

If the first complaint mentioned is not necessarily the most important, why do we behave as if it is the only one likely to be offered? We all can recall consultations that have suffered from this approach with the real problem concerning the patient surfacing very late in the interview after the precious allotted time has been used on a less important topic. Sometimes it is even worse: we may not discover the main reason for the consultation at all and the interview ends without the patient plucking up courage to mention their second, more important agenda item.

How can we overcome this problem? How do we make a route plan of the consultation rather than blindly setting off down the first road that we come across? Here, we discuss three related skills that can help the doctor understand not only why the patient has come but also as many as possible of the issues that they wish to discuss and their relative importance:

1 the opening question
2 listening
3 screening and agenda setting.

The opening question

NEW CONSULTATIONS

Near to the beginning of the interview, it is important to ask the patient an open question such as *'What would you like to discuss today?'*. We all tend to have a favourite stock question that we use repeatedly; here are some examples of phrases that participants attending our courses say they use time and time again:

- *'How can I help?'*
- *'Tell me what you have come to see me about.'*
- *'What would you like to talk about today?'*
- *'What can I do for you?'*
- *'How are you doing?'*
- *'How are things?'*
- *'What's up?'*
- *'Fine, so, off you go ...'*
- *Nothing said (all implied in body language).*

The exact words that we use can become a mantra that we repeat without thought. But, in fact, the phrasing of this simple task can make a considerable difference to the nature of the remaining interview. The format of the question used can subtly change the type of response that the patient provides.

More general enquiries such as *'How are you doing?'* allow the patient to state in broad terms how they are feeling but might not discover the actual problem that they have come about. *'I'm fine but my arthritis is terrible at the moment'* might be the response although the patient has actually come to discuss worsening migraines. This ambiguity might be apparent to a specialist neurologist but not to a general internist who does not have such a focused territory. The doctor needs to be aware of the type of question that he has asked and not assume the reason for the visit until he has asked a more specific follow-up: *'Is that why you have come to see me this morning?'*.

'How can I help you?' is more explicit, implying you want to know what the patient wishes to discuss today, although it might limit the patient to medical matters that the doctor can 'help' with.

'Tell me what you have come to see me about' is less medical, more open and might signal your willingness to listen to a wider agenda.

'What's on your agenda today?' certainly implies that you would like to encourage the patient to make a list of all the problems they would like to discuss, but might not be understood by all patients.

'Fine', *'yes'* or using body language alone and saying nothing at all are extremely open methods of starting and giving the patient the floor, but give little initial direction to the patient as to whether to tell you about one problem in great detail or list all of the problems.

We are not suggesting that there is one correct opening method to be used on all occasions. However, there is clearly a need for doctors to raise their awareness and think more carefully about the consequences of how they start each consultation.

FOLLOW-UP VISITS

Follow-up visits have much more in common with new consultations than is often believed. The key here is not to make the assumption that you know the reason for the visit until you have actually asked the patient. It is so easy to assume that the patient has come for their routine check and move straight into *'How are you getting along with your new pills?'* when in fact the patient has a more pressing or at least a second agenda to discuss. Yet it can sound as if you do not remember the patient at all if you start, as in a new appointment, with *'What would you like to discuss today?'*. Perhaps instead you might start with your understanding of the reason for the visit, as in *'Am I right in thinking that you have come for your routine check'?* or *'I've come to see how you're doing and check your incision'*, and then ask the patient to confirm by adding *'Is there anything else you would like to talk about today as well?'*.

Listening to the patient's opening statement

LEARNING HOW TO LISTEN AT THE BEGINNING OF THE CONSULTATION IS THE FIRST STEP TO AN EFFICIENT AND ACCURATE CONSULTATION

It seems at first glance that giving the patient time, space and encouragement to have the floor while the doctor deliberately sits back and listens might not be the most efficient way of beginning an interview. Often, doctors are under so much pressure from time constraints that they feel the need to force the pace by quickly moving into questioning mode and taking the initiative. Yet this approach so often leads doctors to explore the first item offered by the patient which, as we have seen, can be counter-productive. So how do we address this problem? How do we establish that listening to the patient early on in the consultation is rewarded by a far more efficient and accurate interview overall?

LISTENING RATHER THAN QUESTIONING ALLOWS DOCTORS AND PATIENTS TO ACHIEVE MORE OF THEIR OBJECTIVES FOR THIS PART OF THE CONSULTATION

Reviewing the objectives for this first part of the consultation helps us to find our bearings. Our objectives fall into three broad categories. The first is to understand what the patient wants to discuss today and to plan with the patient how to approach the rest of the consultation. The second is to make the patient feel comfortable, welcomed and an important part of the proceedings, to establish initial rapport. The third is to gauge how the patient is feeling, to be aware of the patient as a person.

How do we achieve all of these simultaneously and with the greatest ease? As we will see in Chapter 3, as soon as the doctor moves into detailed questioning, the patient tends to become a passive contributor. The doctor has to follow each closed question with another, his mind is forced away from the patient's responses into diagnostic reasoning and the interview prematurely focuses on one particular area. In contrast, following an open-ended initial statement or question with attentive listening allows the doctor to discover more of the patient's agenda, to hear the story from the patient's perspective, to appear supportive and interested and, by concentrating on the patient, to pick up cues to their feelings and emotional state that could otherwise be missed.

WHAT IS THE EVIDENCE TO SUPPORT LISTENING?

The importance of doctor's listening skills at the beginning of the consultation has been beautifully demonstrated by two of the most quoted papers in the communication literature, those of Beckman and Frankel (1984) and Beckman *et al.* (1985).

We have known for a long time, from Byrne and Long's work in primary care (1976), that many dysfunctional consultations arise because of difficulties in discovering why the patient has come. One of the problems lies with the patient's tendency to withhold psychosocial and other important concerns until later in the visit when they have tested the water and gained confidence in the doctor. Anxiety or embarrassment about a symptom or a serious worry might make the patient delay mentioning it until late in the day. These late announcements have been termed 'hidden agendas' (Barsky 1981).

This approach to thinking about the interview focuses attention on the patient's decision to withhold, delay or share information. However, more recent research has concentrated on the role that the doctor plays. It has looked at the influence that a doctor's behaviour has on the placement and flow of information provided by the patient and has discovered that doctors' own words and actions have a startling effect on whether (or when) they discover the full reasons for the patient's attendance. Doctors' behaviour may well be more influential here than patients'.

Byrne and Long (1976) showed that many doctors are not good listeners and have fixed routines of interviewing patients which demonstrate little capacity for variation to meet an individual patient's needs. In their key research, Beckman and Frankel (1984) have taken this further by analysing exactly how a doctor's use of words and questions can so easily and inadvertently direct the patient away from disclosing their reasons for wishing to see the doctor. A host of revealing facts was uncovered by their research:

- doctors frequently interrupted patients before they had completed their opening statement – after a mean time of only 18 seconds!
- only 23% of patients completed their opening statement
- in only one out of 51 interrupted statements was the patient allowed to complete their opening statement later
- 94% of all interruptions concluded with the doctor obtaining the floor
- the longer the doctor waited before interruption, the more complaints were elicited
- allowing the patient to complete the opening statement led to a significant reduction in late-arising problems
- clarifying or closed questions were the most frequent cause of interruption but any utterance by the doctor that specifically encouraged the patient to give further information about

any one problem could also cause disruption: this, perhaps surprisingly, included echoing of the patient's words

- in 34 out of 51 visits, the doctor interrupted the patient after the initial concern, apparently assuming that the first complaint was the chief one
- the serial order in which the patients presented their problems was not related to their clinical importance
- most patients who were allowed to complete their opening statement without interruption took less than 60 seconds and none took longer than 150 seconds, even when encouraged to continue.

Beckman and Frankel have shown us that it is the early pursuit, by closed questioning, of the first problem mentioned that prevents doctors from discovering all the issues that a patient wishes to discuss. The emphasis quickly shifts from a patient-centred to a physician-centred format. Once this is done, the patient tends to remain in a more passive role, trying to comply by giving short answers, perhaps assuming that if the competent doctor needs to know something he will ask. Inefficient and inaccurate information gathering ensues. Not only does the interview steam ahead before the main concern has necessarily been discovered but hypothesis testing proceeds without patients having a chance to tell their story or to provide information which closed questioning may never discover.

Beckman and Frankel clearly demonstrate that even minimal interruptions to patients' initial statements can actually prevent other concerns from appearing at all or can make important complaints arise late in the consultation. By asking patients to tell you more about any one problem, you restrict their options, preventing them from expanding on other information that they would like to tell you. The patient is in fact faced with a practical problem when the doctor moves in with an interruption. Say the patient has mentioned headaches but is interrupted before they can mention their recent palpitations and marital problems. 'Tell me more about your headaches' or, worse, 'Where do you get the pain?' restricts the discussion to the headaches and limits both the patient's options and the efficiency of the interview as a whole.

Wissow et al. (1994) have since shown that paediatricians' use of attentive listening is positively associated with parents' disclosure of psychosocial problems while Putnam et al. (1988) have shown that it is possible to teach medical residents the skills of attentive listening and that such teaching leads to a significant increase in patient exposition without any associated increase in the length of the interview.

WHAT ARE THE SPECIFIC SKILLS OF ATTENTIVE LISTENING?

Listening is often equated with 'sitting and doing nothing', a passive rather than active approach. Yet, as Egan (1990) says in *The Skilled Helper*:

How many times have you heard someone exclaim, 'You're not listening to what I'm saying!'. When the person accused of not listening answers, 'I am too; I can repeat everything you've said', the accuser is not comforted. What people look for in attending and listening is not the other person's ability to repeat their words. A tape recorder would do that perfectly. People want more than physical presence in human communication; they want the other person to be present psychologically, socially and emotionally.

In fact, attentive listening is both active and highly skilled. There are four specific skill areas that can help us to develop our ability to listen attentively:

1 wait time
2 facilitative response
3 non-verbal skills
4 picking up verbal and non-verbal cues.

1 *Wait time*. Making the shift from speaking to listening at appropriate moments in the consultation is not easy. Inadvertently, we often find ourselves preparing our next question rather than focusing attention on what the patient is saying. We may become so involved in formulating our next question that we divert our own attention from hearing their message and, by interrupting, fail to give the patient adequate time to respond. Evidence from the world of education rather than medicine helps to illuminate the value to both doctor and patient of allowing the patient more space to think before answering or to go on after pausing.

Over a period of 20 years, Rowe (1986) studied non-medical teachers in a wide variety of classroom settings. She found that when teachers asked questions they waited one second or less for a reply. Similarly, they only waited one second after a student stopped speaking before they responded. However, if the teachers were trained to increase their pauses at each of these key points to three seconds, remarkable changes occurred in the students' behaviour in class. The students contributed more often, spoke for longer, asked more questions, provided more evidence for their thinking and failed to respond less often. Difficult or 'invisible' students started to contribute successfully. In turn, teachers asked their students fewer questions but of a more flexible nature, and they increased their expectations of their students.

In the medical interview, using wait time effectively allows the patient time to think and to contribute more without being interrupted and the doctor to have time to listen, think and respond more flexibly.

2 *Facilitative response*. Some doctors clearly have a greater ability than others to encourage their patients to say more about a topic, to indicate to patients that they are interested in what they are saying and that they would like them to continue. This is often achieved very efficiently with minimal or no interruption and it is worth considering exactly what these minimal cues are that seem to be such powerful indicators to patients that we are listening and wish to hear.

We will look in more detail at facilitation skills in Chapter 3, but at this point we would like to consider which specific facilitative responses are of value in this opening phase of the consultation. Research has clearly shown that the skills employed in attentive listening are different at different stages in the consultation and that facilitation skills known to be helpful later on in the consultation are in fact counter-productive when used early on in the interview.

Beckman and Frankel's (1984) work provides clear guidance here. Their work looked specifically at which facilitative interventions by physicians allowed patients to continue and complete their initial statement of concerns and which interrupted the patient, promoted premature exploration of one specific area and prevented the physician from discovering more of the concerns that the patient wished to discuss. They showed that repetition (echoing), paraphrasing and interpretation, which are all valuable facilitative skills later on in the interview, potentially act as interrupters at the beginning of the interview whereas other, more neutral facilitative phrases such as *'uh-huh'*, *'go on'*, *'yes'*, *'um'*, *'I see'* serve to encourage the patient to continue along their own path.

3 *Non-verbal skills.* We provide a more detailed exploration of non-verbal skills when we look at 'Building the relationship' in Chapter 4. Here, however, we would like to highlight some issues about non-verbal communication that are particularly relevant to the beginning of the consultation.

Much of our willingness to listen is signalled through our non-verbal behaviour which immediately gives the patient strong cues as to our level of interest in them and in their problems. Many individual components are involved in non-verbal communication, including posture, movement, proximity, direction of gaze, eye contact, gestures, affect, vocal cues (tone, rate, volume of speech), facial expression, touch, physical appearance and environmental cues (placement of furniture, lighting, warmth). All these skills can assist in demonstrating attentiveness to patients and facilitate the formation of a supportive relationship; in contrast, ineffective attending behaviour both closes off the interaction and prohibits relationship building (Gazda *et al.* 1995).

Among the most important of all the non-verbal skills is eye contact. We can so easily be distracted from providing this by the records or the computer as we grapple to comprehend our patient's problem; yet, poor eye contact can be readily misinterpreted by the patient as lack of interest and can inhibit open communication. First impressions are very important here.

Communication research has shown that non-verbal messages tend to override verbal messages when the two are inconsistent or contradictory (Koch 1971; McCroskey *et al.* 1971). If you provide the verbal message that you want the patient to tell you all about their problem while at the same time you speak quickly, look harassed and avoid eye contact, your non-verbal message will usually win out. The patient will correctly construe that time is at a premium today and may not tell you about the problem in sufficient detail.

The importance of both verbal and non-verbal facilitative responses lies in the message that they impart to the patient. One of the principles of communication that we outlined in Chapter 1 concerned reducing uncertainty and establishing mutually understood common ground. Facilitative responses are effective in encouraging patients to tell their story because they directly signal to patients something about our intentions and attitude towards them and interest in their story. In the absence of these skills, the patient remains uncertain about our interest in what they are saying and our need for them to continue with their account: we might be clear in our own minds that we wish the interview to proceed in a certain way but is our verbal and non-verbal behaviour skilful enough for the patient to share that understanding?

4 *Picking up verbal and non-verbal cues.* Another important skill of attentive listening is that of picking up patients' verbal and non-verbal cues. This requires both listening and observation. Often, patients' ideas, concerns and expectations are expressed in non-verbal cues and indirect comments rather than overt statements (Tuckett *et al.* 1985). These cues often feature very early in the patient's exposition of their problems and the doctor needs to look out specifically for them from the very beginning of the interview. The danger lies in either missing these messages altogether or assuming we know what they mean without checking them out with the patient either now or later in the interview.

WHAT ARE THE ADVANTAGES OF ATTENTIVE LISTENING?

Full attention through active listening allows you to:

- signal your interest to the patient
- hear their story
- prevent yourself from making premature hypotheses and chasing down blind alleys
- reduce late-arising complaints
- hear both 'disease' and 'illness', as discussed in Chapter 3
- not think of the next question (which blocks your listening and renders the patient passive)
- calibrate the patient's emotional state
- observe more carefully and pick up verbal and non-verbal cues.

With so much to hear and see at the beginning of the interview, why not consciously set aside the first minute or two for the patient and concentrate on listening and facilitating rather than questioning? Listening attentively instead of moving immediately to a series of questions about the history allows us to achieve more of our objectives – although it requires very little time, using these early moments of the consultation wisely pays off handsomely.

Screening

In the discussion above, we have seen how using an appropriate opening question combined with attentive listening and specific facilitation skills allows the physician to discover more of the patient's agenda in the early part of the consultation. Now, we would like to explore how making a further deliberate attempt to discover all of the patient's problem *before* actively exploring any one of them can further increase the accuracy and efficiency of consultations.

Screening is the process of deliberately checking with the patient that you have discovered all that they wish to discuss by asking further open-ended enquiries. Rather than assuming that the patient has mentioned all their difficulties, double-check:

'So you've been getting headaches and dizziness lately. Has anything else been bothering you?'

If the patient continues, resume listening until the patient stops again; then repeat the screening process until eventually the patient says that they have finished:

'So you've also been feeling very tired and irritable and were wondering if you might be anaemic. Anything else at all?'

At the end of this process when the patient says *'No, that's about it'*, you might wish to confirm your understanding and give the patient an opportunity to know what you have heard:

'So, as I understand it, you've been getting headaches and dizziness but have also been feeling tired, rather irritable and a bit low, and your concern is that you might be anaemic. Did I get that right?'

Often, this method of checking reveals symptoms and concerns relating to the initial complaint, but the patient might not yet have revealed a totally separate problem. You might wish to perform one last check here:

'I can see these symptoms must have been worrying you and we'll need to explore them further. Before we do, let me just check whether there are any other areas that you hope I might be able to help you with today as well.'

The patient might then produce a second problem area, *'Well, I've also got this terrible cough'* or a social problem, *'Well, I'm really terribly worried about my daughter'*. Without this check, you might only discover these issues at the end of the consultation and not have any time or patience left to deal with them.

The four-part approach to identifying the patient's agenda:

1 opening question
2 listening
3 screening
4 confirming

offers many advantages to the doctor and the patient over the more traditional alternative of:

1 asking
2 assuming
3 proceeding.

For the doctor, there is a better chance of discovering the patient's full agenda, negotiating how best to use the time available and pacing the interview appropriately. Screening also provides a way for doctors to check out their expectations and assumptions about why the patient may have come or what they want to talk about, helping the doctor to keep an open mind.

For the patient, there is the reassurance that you are really interested in their problems and thoughts: this in turn enhances trust and disclosure. Helping the patient reveal their most important problems early on prevents the patient's attention from remaining focused on how and when to introduce their unstated concern rather than on the agenda in progress (Korsch *et al.* 1968; Mehrabian and Ksionsky 1974). Screening helps prevent uncertainty in the patient's mind leading to distraction and blocking effective communication.

Patients may of course still reveal an additional or temporarily forgotten problem, or a hidden agenda, later in the interview, perhaps when they have tested the water and gained confidence in the relationship. Screening encourages but does not guarantee early problem identification and so we must still remain open to late-arising complaints and be sensitive to the reasons the patient might have for delaying their introduction.

Several North American teaching texts propose the following sequence for the early part of the consultation (Riccardi and Kurtz 1983; Lipkin 1987; Cohen-Cole 1991):

- encourage the patient to disclose their main concerns by attentive listening without interruption or premature closure
- confirm the list identified so far by summarizing
- check repeatedly for additional concerns – *'Is there anything else you wish to discuss today?'* – until the patient indicates that there are none
- negotiate an agenda for the consultation.

We look more closely at the skills of checking and summarizing in Chapter 3.

THE BALANCE BETWEEN LISTENING AND SCREENING

Having discovered the importance of screening for the full range of problems, learners often identify a dilemma about when exactly to screen and when to listen. A balance is necessary in the use of these two complementary skills which will be determined in part by the context of each interview.

In certain interviews, it is possible and beneficial to be quite up front about screening and to explain your plan to the patient right from the start. So, as an example, the patient referred to a specialist might receive the following introduction:

'Hello, I'm Dr Smith. I've got a letter from your GP so I've some idea of why you've come today, but I'd like to hear the story from you, first hand, and then try to help as best I can. I'd like to start, if you agree, with us making a list of all the problems you've been having or things you'd like help with and then we can explore them together in more detail.'

This approach makes the structure very clear to the patient and makes it apparent that the doctor wants to understand the whole of their agenda from the start and will then attend to each of their concerns. Otherwise, the patient may not know if they are expected to steam ahead with one problem or to mention them all briefly.

At the other extreme, a patient who enters the room and immediately breaks into a story that they clearly need to tell, or a patient who on sitting down dissolves into tears because her father has just died, deserves our full attention now: here, listening takes priority over screening. It would be inappropriate to interrupt and say 'We'll come back to that. Is there anything else that you would like to discuss today?'!

Some patients come with a pre-written list, giving the doctor a perfect opportunity to screen the agenda and negotiate what is possible in the time today. Other patients come with a well-rehearsed speech that they have nervously prepared: the telling of it is essential for the patient's peace of mind before the doctor and patient can settle down to work together. Often, this opening statement can be so rich in feelings, thoughts, ideas, concerns and expectations and give such clues to the patient's lifeworld that it would be a mistake not to give the patient the floor to express their story. If you do not listen first, you might well miss clues that could be important in helping the patient with their problem.

This dilemma can be resolved by another of the principles of communication that we have already discussed – *dynamism*. What is appropriate for one situation is inappropriate for another and we have to continually monitor how best to approach the consultation as we proceed. Knowing that it is helpful to both listen and screen and being flexible enough to use both appropriately in differing situations is the key.

Agenda setting

Screening naturally leads on to negotiating and setting an agenda, taking both the patient's and the doctor's needs into account. In keeping with our emphasis on developing a partnership between patient and physician – a collaborative relationship – this is an overt and involving approach to clarifying how the interview should proceed.

We look in more detail at how to structure an interview in Chapter 3 when we consider summary and signposting. We will describe how these methods enhance the doctor's ability to consider where he has got to so far in the interview, what exactly he is trying to achieve next and how to verbalize these thoughts to the patient. There are many advantages to this over simply steaming ahead without explaining the process to the patient. For the doctor, organization of thought prevents aimless or unnecessary questioning and incomplete data gathering. For the patient, the structure of the interview is made overt and an opportunity is provided for more involvement and more responsibility in what is taking place.

Agenda setting is another example of structuring the consultation. Priorities can be established and negotiated:

'Shall we start with the new problem, the diarrhoea, and then move onto the problems you have been having with your medication?'

The doctor's agenda can also be added:

'OK, let's think about your headaches and then look at the rash. I wouldn't mind checking on your blood pressure and your thyroid pills too later on, if that's all right.'

Problems with time can be acknowledged and negotiated:

'That's quite a list for us to get through and I'm not sure that we are going to have enough time to do it all justice. How about …?'

In negotiating priorities, a balance may need to be struck between the patient's personal hierarchy of concerns and the doctor's medical understanding of which problems might be more immediately important:

'I can see that the arthritis is the thing that's really bothering you most today but if you don't mind, I'd rather we started by checking out those chest pains you had last week.'

Interestingly, Levinson *et al.* (1997) showed that primary care physicians who educated the patient about what to expect and the flow of the visit were less likely to have suffered malpractice claims.

Notice that in agenda setting and negotiating you are not just telling the patient what you are going to do but are inviting the patient to participate in making an agreed plan. One of the principles of communication that we discussed in Chapter 1 was that *effective communication promotes an interaction rather than a process of direct transmission.* Cassata (1978) explained how crystallizing agendas at the beginning of the consultation promotes just such an interaction, a two-way communication that encourages the patient to be a more active, responsible and autonomous participant throughout the consultation. Another of our five principles concerns *reducing uncertainty.* Here, overt agenda setting does just that by establishing mutually understood common ground. Joos *et al.* (1996) provide research which validates this approach. They taught internal medicine residents and physicians the skills of eliciting the patient's full concerns and negotiating a mutually agreed agenda; they demonstrated that doctors who received this training not only subsequently discovered more of their patients' concerns but, equally importantly, achieved this without any increase in the length of the visit.

Summary

In this chapter, we have examined the skills of initiating the consultation, one of the most important parts of any interview. The skills involved in establishing initial rapport, identifying the issues that the patient wishes to discuss and agreeing on an agenda set the scene for the rest of the interview. They directly influence whether the three goals of medical communication, *accuracy, efficiency and supportiveness*, are achieved throughout the interview as a whole.

The skills of initiation are very different from the skills of gathering information, as we have shown in the *Calgary–Cambridge observation guide*. Yet so often we do not separate out these tasks in our minds and they merge together with deleterious results. Clearly, having in mind a structure for the consultation as we progress through the interview is of vital importance. Before going on to explore the patient's problems in detail, it is helpful to ask 'Have I achieved my objectives for this first part of the interview – have I established a supportive environment; have I discovered all the problems that the patient has come to discuss; have I developed a mutually agreed plan for the consultation; have I enabled the patient to become part of a collaborative process?' Once these tasks have been completed, the doctor can then move on to gathering information about each problem.

3

Gathering information

Introduction

Having seen how vital the beginning of the interview is to successful doctor–patient communication, we now turn our attention to the next section of the interview – gathering information.

For many years, we have recognized the overriding importance of history taking to diagnosis. Clinical studies have shown repeatedly that the history contributes 60–80% of the data for diagnosis (Hampton *et al.* 1975; Sandler 1980; Kassirer 1983; Peterson *et al.* 1992): in Hampton's study in medical out-patients, the history alone was sufficient to make the diagnosis in 66 out of 80 patients. Yet the way that many doctors have been taught to take a history in medical school can lead to inaccuracy and inefficiency. Traditional questioning methods do not encourage comprehensive history taking or effective hypothesis generation. Fortunately, recent developments in communication theory and research have greatly improved our understanding of the *process* of gathering information. They have also opened up a whole new *content* area of history taking, namely the patient's perspective of their illness (McWhinney 1989). Traditional medical interviewing has concentrated on pathological disease at the expense of understanding the highly individual needs of each patient. As a consequence, much of the information required to understand our patients' problems remains hidden. Studies of patient satisfaction, adherence, recall and physiological outcome all validate the need for a broader view of history taking that encompasses the patient's lifeworld as well as the doctor's more focused biological perspective.

Problems in communication

There is considerable evidence of communication problems in the gathering information phase of the consultation.

- Byrne and Long's (1976) classic work studying 2000 consultations in British primary care showed that doctors used a remarkably uniform style despite differences in the problems presented to them or in their patients' behaviour. They often pursued a 'doctor-centred', closed approach to information gathering that discouraged patients from telling their story or voicing their concerns.

- Platt and McMath (1979) observed 300 encounters in hospital internal medicine in the USA and showed that both a 'high control style' and premature focus on medical problems lead to an over-narrow approach to hypothesis generation and to limitation of the patient's ability to communicate their concerns. These in turn lead to inaccurate consultations.
- Tuckett et al.'s (1985) research on information giving in British general practice, which we will explore more fully in Chapter 5, demonstrated the central importance of eliciting patients' beliefs about their illness in enabling patients to understand and recall information. Yet their research efforts were hampered by the very few examples that they were able to find of doctors asking patients to volunteer their ideas or even of doctors asking patients to elaborate on their ideas if they did spontaneously bring them up.
- Kleinman et al. (1978) used cross-cultural work to show how undiscovered discordance between the health beliefs of patient and physician can lead to problems in patient satisfaction, adherence, management and outcome.
- Maguire and Rutter (1976) showed serious deficiencies in senior medical students' information-gathering skills: few students managed to discover the patient's main problem, clarify the exact nature of the problem and explore ambiguous statements, clarify with precision, elicit the impact of the problem on daily life, respond to verbal cues, cover more personal topics or use facilitation. Most used closed, lengthy, multiple and repetitive questions.

A theoretical discussion of information gathering

Before we look at the objectives and skills involved in this part of the medical interview, we would like to explore two contrasting theoretical concepts of information gathering – the traditional method of history taking and the disease–illness model.

The traditional method of history taking

The traditional method of history taking is so firmly established in medical practice that it is easy to assume that it is the correct approach. Yet often in medicine we make such assumptions without considering the origins of what we do and their relevance to modern-day practice. McWhinney (1989) has eloquently traced the origins, strengths and weaknesses of the traditional clinical method which we briefly précis here.

ORIGINS OF THE TRADITIONAL METHOD

At the beginning of the nineteenth century, a new method of clinical medicine began to emerge, pioneered in post-revolutionary France. Prior to this, medicine had lacked any scientific basis: patients' symptoms had been the focus of doctors' attention and there had been little understanding of underlying disease processes. Innovations such as the stethoscope now revealed a whole new range of clinical information. At the same time, physicians began to examine the internal organs after death and tried to correlate physical signs in life to post-mortem findings in death. From this point on, the physical expression of the patient's illness became central to the profession's approach: it became the aim of the diagnostician to interpret the patient's symptoms in terms of specific diseases and to provide a scientific explanation. This change was to herald the incredible advances in diagnosis and treatment of the twentieth century.

By 1880, a fully defined clinical method had become established. This is apparent from hospital clinical records where the structured method of recording the history and examination that we are all so familiar with today had already taken root (Tait 1979). The history of present complaint, history of past illness, drug and allergy history, family history, personal and social history and functional enquiry provided a standard method of recording clinical enquiries and forged an ordered approach to history taking.

This method still dominates medicine today and has been consolidated by the incorporation of powerful new methods of investigation which have further enhanced our ability to interpret the patient's illness in terms of underlying physical pathology. Imaging, microbiology, biochemistry and haematology are the essentials of our trade: they have taken our understanding of the disease process to the cellular level and beyond.

STRENGTHS

It is the scientific approach to the patient that is the traditional clinical method's greatest strength. There is no doubt that the development of a method of classification of the underlying cause of disease paved the way for the advances in medical science that have followed. It provided the first real possibility of precise clinical audit with the pathologist giving clinicians feedback on their diagnostic skills. It gave a common language to unify the 'medical approach'.

It also provided physicians with a clear method of taking and recording the clinical history, supplying a carefully structured template with which to arrive at a diagnosis or exclude physical disease. It simplified and unified a very complex process, prevented the omission of key points and enabled the data extracted from the patient to appear in a standard assimilatable form.

WEAKNESSES

The strength of the traditional clinical method is also its weakness. As the profession has embraced the objectivity required to diagnose disease in terms of underlying pathology, it has increasingly concentrated on the individual parts of the body that are malfunctioning and has honed this process down to a cellular and now molecular level. Yet this very detached objectivity so easily overlooks the patient as a whole. As Cassell (1985) put it, 'The patient's individual concerns are brushed aside to support the function of their organs'.

The scientific method does not aim to understand the meaning of the illness for the patient or place it in the context of his life and family. Subjective matters such as beliefs, anxieties and concerns are not the remit of the traditional approach: science deals with the objective, that which can be measured, whereas the patient's feelings, thoughts and concerns are unquantifiable and subjective and therefore are deemed less worthy of consideration.

Medical students have been traditionally brought up in this world of the objective and the technological: at the expense of understanding the sick person, they have been taught to concentrate on the underlying disease mechanism and thereby to avoid the patient's perceptions and feelings. Unsupervised and undervalued forays into the uncharted territory of the patient's ideas and emotions only serve to reinforce the need for objectivity.

There is a further problem with the classic method of history taking. The way that doctors have been taught to ask specific closed questions about each symptom suggests that if they ask the 15 questions that they have been taught about the functioning of a particular organ system, they will gather all the information required to make a diagnosis. But as we shall see later, this closed approach to questioning is by itself an inefficient and inaccurate method of history taking which does not promote effective information gathering (Evans *et al.* 1991). In fact, it is the premature search for scientific facts that stops us from listening, that both prevents us from taking an accurate history and from picking up the cues to patients' problems and concerns. Disease-centred medicine can so quickly turn into doctor-centred medicine to the detriment of us all.

The disease–illness model

McWhinney (1989) and his colleagues at the University of Western Ontario proposed a 'transformed clinical method' to replace the traditional method of history taking. This approach, which requires doctors to understand their patients as well as their patients' diseases, has also been called 'patient-centred clinical interviewing' to differentiate it from the 'doctor-centred' approach that attempts to interpret the patients' illnesses only from the traditional perspective of disease and pathology (Stewart *et al.* 1995).

Patient-centred medicine encourages doctors to consider both the doctor's and patient's perspectives and agendas in each interview (Mischler 1984; Campion *et al.* 1992; Keller and Carroll 1994). The disease–illness model (Fig. 3.1) provides a practical way of using these ideas in everyday clinical practice.

DEFINITION OF DISEASE AND ILLNESS

The beauty of this analysis of gathering information is the clarity with which it demonstrates how doctors need to explore both 'disease' and 'illness' to fulfil their unique role as medical practitioners. 'Disease' is the biomedical cause of sickness in terms of pathophysiology. Clearly it is the doctor's role to search for symptoms and signs of underlying disease. Discovering a diagnosis for the patient's 'disease' is the doctor's traditional and central agenda. 'Illness', in contrast, is the individual patient's unique experience of sickness, how each patient perceives, experiences and copes with their illness. The patient's perspective is not as narrow as the doctor's and includes the feelings, thoughts, concerns and effect on life that any episode of sickness induces. It represents the patient's response to events around him, his understanding of what is happening to him and his expectations of help.

Patients can be ill but have no disease. Often we cannot find a root cause for symptoms in any underlying pathological disease. For example, consider the patient with a bereavement reaction and the symptoms that grief can produce; or the businessman with tension headaches; or the young child with problems at school leading to abdominal pain. On the other hand patients can have a disease but not be knowingly ill, for example asymptomatic disease such as ovarian cancer or hypertension.

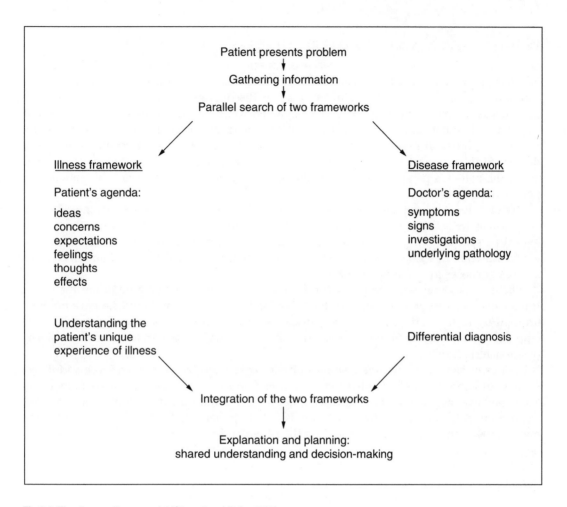

Fig 3.1 The disease–illness model (Stewart and Roter 1989).

Disease and illness normally coexist but one of the great fascinations of medicine is how the same disease causes remarkably different illness experiences in each individual. Imagine for a moment all the patients you have seen with any one condition. The variation between each patient's reaction to their similar symptoms or to their common diagnosis is enormous. Their thoughts, feelings, ideas, concerns, expectations, support systems and previous life experiences influence not only their ability to cope but also the physical effect of the disease itself. One person with a sore throat is happy to wait for nature to provide a cure and does not go to the doctor at all while another wants antibiotics because he remembers how awful it was when he had quinsy. One woman with breast cancer presents with a tiny lump; another is discovered by chance to have a hidden fungating mass.

WHY DO DOCTORS NEED TO EXPLORE BOTH PERSPECTIVES?

Doctors have always attempted to separate out these two contrasting perspectives of sickness but in the past have tended to discard the patient's illness framework as simply a collection of confounding variables which get in the way of discovering the underlying diagnosis. A patient's fear, anxiety and pain threshold can all encroach on the doctor's ability to find out, say, if an abdominal pain is appendicitis or not. Doctors may only consider the patient's unique response in order to prevent it from clouding their technological judgement. All too often doctors focus only on the disease itself, discard the understanding that they have obtained about the patient's perspective of their illness and thereby fail to consider the patient as a person (Cassell 1985).

Mischler (1984) has explained how the doctor, in his desperation to make a diagnosis, selectively listens to patients' comments that help him interpret their problems from the technological perspective. He does not hear or pursue comments that give him insight into their world. Mischler describes this as 'two parallel monologues' in which patient and doctor talk at cross purposes in different languages.

Whereas doctors have discarded the information that they have obtained from the illness framework, healers, practitioners of alternative medicine and counsellors who have not been brought up in the tradition of Western disease-centred medicine have tended to place less emphasis on information from the disease framework and have concentrated instead on 'illness' (Kleinman *et al.* 1978).

Doctors in fact have a unique responsibility to do both, to listen to the disease and illness frameworks and not discard either (Smith and Hoppe 1991). The disease–illness model does not in any way negate the scientific disease approach but adds a patient-centred arm as well. Doctors are not counsellors whose sole aim is to help patients to become aware of how their own thoughts and feelings are influencing their lives and their illness; doctors have the extra responsibility and burden of diagnosing and treating disease. But if they consider their role as purely that of discovering disease, they will not fully help their patients, each of whom has very individual needs.

Doctors need to take into account both their own traditional disease agenda and the patient's very personal illness agenda. When a patient presents with joint pains, the doctor may see his role in terms of diagnosis and treatment of any underlying disease. But the patient's main concern may be the possibility of loss of future independence – her agenda may concern discussing prognosis more than diagnosis. These two agendas overlap but without addressing the patient's beliefs and concerns as well as diagnosing the disease process, the doctor will not have fully served the patient as an individual. The patient-centred approach enlarges the doctor's agenda to take account of both disease and illness.

The advantages of taking a history that includes both arms of the disease–illness model are numerous:

Supporting, understanding and building a relationship. Taking only a traditional, disease-centred history of chest pain in a 55-year-old man may well allow you to diagnose angina and plan investigation and treatment. While this is an absolutely necessary task, failing to understand the meaning of the chest pain to the patient and the implications that your diagnosis might have for that individual may well limit your effectiveness as a doctor. The patient may become agitated at the mention of angina as his father died suddenly from a heart attack at the same age. Or he may have been very fit and active up until now and be devastated that heart disease might prevent the active future he had planned. He may be a commercial traveller whose livelihood depends on his ability to drive. His wife may be ill and he might not want to burden her with his problems. Your capacity to help him depends on your ability not only to diagnose effectively but also to understand your patient's perspective and support him through adversity.

The traditional disease model does not explain everything about a patient's problems. There may not be a 'disease' in terms of the traditional medical model to explain our 55-year-old man's chest pain and his feelings of illness. It may have roots in personal unhappiness, in stress at home or at work, in anxiety about health. Although it is clearly the doctor's responsibility to exclude physical disease, however hard they try doctors will not find a disease in all their patients. Even if they do, it may not explain why the patient has come to see the doctor on this occasion; a muscular pain may well be tolerated when the patient is comfortable with his life but be cause for concern when the patient is under stress.

We need to extend medical interviewing to include not only the disease but also the illness framework. Using just the disease approach, our man's chest pain may not sound ischaemic and his ECG may be normal. But if he keeps returning with unexplained pain, we may feel forced to investigate further. Exploring the illness perspective as well may allow him to talk about his marital difficulties or his unresolved grief which in itself may well lead to resolution of his symptoms. Searching both frameworks can make the consultation more accurate and efficient as well as supportive: in Stewart *et al.*'s (1997) recent study in family practice, patient centredness and the patient's perception of finding common ground regarding both frameworks resulted in fewer follow-up appointments, fewer investigations and fewer referrals.

There is considerable research evidence to support the failure of organic disease to explain many patients' problems. In 50% of patients presenting to general practitioners with chest pain, the cause was unproven after six months follow-up (Blacklock 1977). Similar statistics are available for tiredness, abdominal pain and headache. But it would be a mistake to think that this is a problem that is restricted to family medicine – what about the globus of ENT or the irritable bowel syndrome of gastroenterology or the non-organic chest pain of cardiology? All specialists see patients whose symptoms are not caused by disease.

Discovering the patient's perspective can aid diagnosis and make for more effective and efficient interviews. Asking for the patient's ideas can aid diagnosis: discovering that the pain started after a fall may be an important clue to the cause of the problem which might otherwise never have been discovered. Discovering that the patient's agenda is simply to obtain a sickness certificate as their back pain is resolving may save time and money by preventing unnecessary disease-centred questioning or uncalled-for prescribing.

Groundwork for explanation and planning. When we explore explanation and planning in Chapter 5, we will look at the research that demonstrates the central importance of eliciting and understanding the patient's unique perspective of their illness to this later stage of the consultation. We will see that without an explanation that addresses patients' individual ideas, expectations and concerns, patients' recall, understanding, satisfaction and compliance are all likely to suffer.

Tuckett *et al.* (1985) have shown that consultations go wrong where there is an incongruity between the patient's and the doctor's explanatory frameworks. Our 55-year-old man with chest pain might well think that he has lung cancer as his friend has recently died from the disease. You might be perfectly happy that it is musculo-skeletal and of no consequence. Unless you have discovered your patient's ideas and explained why you think that it is not due to cancer, he may leave the consulting room with the nagging doubt that you may not have considered the possibility. This doubt may block the patient's understanding and commitment to your explanations and undermine his acceptance of your diagnosis. Similarly, an elderly woman with arthritis of the knee may not wish any active treatment for a pain that she can easily tolerate – her concern may be that she is developing rheumatoid arthritis like her mother and she might just want reassurance that she is not. Without understanding her expectations, the doctor might use the word arthritis and not explain the difference between osteo- and rheumatoid arthritis. He might prescribe an anti-inflammatory drug which the patient does not wish to take. It is so easy to treat the disease rather than the patient.

So, as well as splitting the two arms of disease and illness apart, the physician has to put the two back together again. This is the stage labelled 'integration' in the disease–illness model. Without this step it is impossible to achieve a shared understanding with the patient about the nature of the problem and its management and difficult to enable the patient to participate in shared decision making.

Basing negotiation on an open understanding of both the doctor's and patient's respective positions and reaching mutually understood common ground is the final aim. But, as we shall see later in this chapter and in Chapter 5, understanding the patient's perspective does not mean abdicating responsibility as doctors and promoting an entirely consumerist approach. Consider the person who attends with a viral sore throat which the doctor thinks does not require antibiotics. Discovering the patient's expectations first rather than assuming that all patients wish to be prescribed antibiotics is helpful in itself. A treatment plan can then be negotiated that is based on a true understanding of the patient's position. Conflict and dissatisfaction can be anticipated and defused. If, as is often the case, the patient would prefer not to have antibiotics if at all possible, a comfortable negotiation is assured from the outset. If, however, they would prefer antibiotics, eliciting and addressing that expectation and explaining your position in relation to their views is vital; only then can the patient understand your rationale and feel their position has at least been taken into consideration.

Objectives

The objectives for the information-gathering part of the interview include:

- exploring and understanding the patient's perspective so as to understand the meaning of the illness for the patient
- exploring the doctor's perspective so as to obtain an adequate 'medical' history
- ensuring that information gathered about both frameworks is accurate, complete and mutually understood
- ensuring that patients feel listened to, that their information and views are welcomed and valued
- continuing to develop a supportive environment and a collaborative relationship
- structuring the consultation to ensure efficient information gathering and to enable the patient to understand and be overtly involved in where the interview is going and why.

Again, these objectives encompass many of the tasks and check-points mentioned in other well-known guides to the consultation:

Byrne and Long (1976)   Phase 3: the doctor conducts a verbal or physical examination or both
                          Phase 4: the doctor or the doctor and the patient or the patient (in that order of probability) consider the condition

Pendleton *et al.* (1984)   To define the reason for the patient's attendance
                          (1) the nature and history of the problems
                          (2) their aetiology
                          (3) the patient's ideas, concerns and expectations
                          (4) the effects of the problems
                          To establish or maintain a relationship with the patient

Neighbour (1987)   Connecting – establishing rapport with the patient
                          Summarizing – 'Have I sufficiently understood why the patient has come to see me?'

Cohen-Cole (1991)   Gathering data to understand the patient's problems
                          Developing rapport and responding to the patient's emotions

Keller and Carroll (1994) Engaging the patient
                          Empathizing with the patient.

'What' to teach and learn about gathering information – the evidence for the skills

Next we examine in detail the individual skills for gathering information listed in Box 3.1 and explore the evidence from theory and research which validates their use in the consultation.

SECTION 1: EXPLORATION OF PROBLEMS

In Chapter 2, we examined the beginning of the interview and saw the advantages of making a route plan of the consultation rather than blindly setting off down the first road that appears. Now we move to the next stage in the consultation where the doctor, after agreeing with the patient on an agenda, wishes to explore each of the patient's problems in turn.

Before looking at the specific skills required to explore a problem area in depth, we examine the central importance of question style to information gathering and in particular, the use of open and closed methods of questioning.

The importance of question style to information gathering

It is easy to assume at this point in the consultation that the doctor's influence on events is limited, that the patient will tell their prepared story, whatever the doctor does or says. But in fact our own actions and utterances profoundly influence our patients' replies and the type of

---

Box 3.1 Skills for gathering information

Exploration of problems

- **Patient's narrative:** encourages patient to tell the story of the problem(s) from when first started to the present in own words (clarifying reason for presenting now)
- **Question style:** uses open and closed questioning techniques, appropriately moving from open-ended to closed
- **Listening:** listens attentively, allowing patient to complete statements without interruption; leaves space for patient to think before answering or go on after pausing
- **Facilitative response:** facilitates patient's responses verbally and non-verbally, e.g. use of encouragement, silence, repetition, paraphrasing, interpretation
- **Clarification:** checks out statements which are vague or need amplification (e.g. 'Could you explain what you mean by light-headed?')
- **Timeframing:** establishing when events in history occurred
- **Internal summary:** periodically summarizes to verify own understanding of what the patient has said; invites patient to correct interpretation and provide further information
- **Language:** uses concise, easily understood questions and comments; avoids or adequately explains jargon

Understanding the patient's perspective

- **Ideas and concerns:** determines patient's (a) ideas (i.e. beliefs) and (b) concerns (including worries) regarding each problem
- **Effects:** determines how each problem affects the patient's life
- **Expectations:** determines patient's goals, what help the patient had expected for each problem
- **Feelings and thoughts:** encourages expression of the patient's feelings and thoughts
- **Cues:** picks up verbal and non-verbal cues (body language, speech, facial expression, affect); checks them out and acknowledges as appropriate

Providing structure to the consultation

- **Internal summary:** summarizes at the end of a specific line of enquiry to confirm understanding before moving on to the next section
- **Signposting:** progresses from one section to another using transitional statements; includes rationale for next section
- **Sequencing:** develops a logical sequence apparent to the patient

responses they provide. How we ask questions plays a central role in the quality and quantity of information that we obtain.

We should remember that as doctors we exert considerable control over the interview. We direct the patient to an area for further exploration and, by the nature of our questions and responses, impose certain limits to the patient's freedom to elaborate. Yet very often we are not consciously aware of the effect that we are having. How can we make this process more intentional so that we can more adeptly choose to use different questioning techniques as and when required? Let us start with some definitions.

WHAT ARE OPEN AND CLOSED QUESTIONS?

Closed (convergent) questions are questions for which a specific and often one-word answer, such as yes or no, is expected. They limit the response to a narrow field set by the questioner: the patient usually provides a response of one or two words without elaboration.

Open (divergent) questioning techniques, in contrast, are designed to introduce an area of enquiry without unduly shaping or focusing the content of the response. They still direct the patient to a specific area but allow the patient more discretion in their answer, suggesting to the patient that elaboration is both appropriate and welcome.

Here are some simple examples of these questioning styles:

Open – *'Tell me about your headaches'*
More specific but still open – *'What makes your headaches better or worse?'*
Closed – *'Do you ever wake up with the headache in the morning?'*

We would like to emphasize that both open and closed questions are valuable. In our efforts to demonstrate that doctors tend to use closed questions too often, at the wrong time and at the expense of open questions, it is all too easy to imply that doctors should not use closed questions at all. Both are essential but achieve very different ends: their use at different times in the interview needs to be chosen with care.

Because asking questions is not the only way to gather information, the term 'question' is something of a misnomer here. More accurate would be the broader open and closed 'questioning techniques'. Many open methods are in fact not questions at all but directive statements:

'Start at the beginning and take me through what has been happening ...'
'Tell me more about that ...'
'Tell me how you have been doing since your operation yesterday ...'

as opposed to questions:

'What has been going on from when you first noticed the pain up until now?
'Why did your doctor admit you to the hospital today?'
'How have you been feeling since your operation ...?'
'What were your thoughts ...?'

WHEN SHOULD WE USE OPEN AND CLOSED METHODS? *THE OPEN-TO-CLOSED CONE*

Understanding how to intentionally choose between open and closed questioning styles at different points in the interview is of key importance. Starting with open questions and later moving to closed questions is called the 'open-to-closed cone' (Goldberg *et al.* 1983). The doctor uses open questioning techniques first to obtain a picture of the problem from the patient's perspective. Later, questioning becomes more focused with increasingly specific though still open questions and eventually closed questions to elicit additional details that the patient may have omitted. The use of open questioning techniques is critical at the beginning of the exploration of any problem; their power as an information-gathering tool here cannot be overemphasized. The most common mistake is to move to closed questioning too quickly.

WHAT ARE THE ADVANTAGES OF OPEN QUESTIONING TECHNIQUES?

Why does staying open before moving to closed questions provide maximum efficiency in information gathering? Look at what might happen if we were to use two very different approaches to the same scenario:

A consultation relying on closed questions might go like this:

Doctor: *'Now about this chest pain – where is the pain?'*
Patient: *'Well, over the front here.'* (pointing to the sternum)
Doctor: *'What are the pains like – are they a dull ache or a sharp pain?'*
Patient: *'Quite sharp really.'*
Doctor: *'Have you taken anything for it?'*
Patient: *'Just some antacids but they don't seem to help much.'*
Doctor: *'Do the pains go anywhere else?'*
Patient: *'No, just there.'*

An initially more open-ended questioning style might reveal very different information:

Doctor: *'Tell me about the chest pain that you have been having.'*
Patient: *'Well, it's been building up over the last few weeks. I've always had a little indigestion but not as bad as this. I get this sharp pain right here* (pointing to sternum) *and then I belch a lot and get a really horrible acid taste in my mouth. It's much worse if I've had a drink or two and I'm not getting much sleep.'*
Doctor: *'I see, can you tell me more about it?'*
Patient: *'Well, I was wondering if it was brought on by the tablets I've been taking for my joints – they've been much worse and I took some ibuprofen. I need to keep going at the moment what with John and all.'*

Why is there such a difference in the information obtained with open questioning?

The advantages of open-questioning methods are that they:

- encourage the patient to tell their story in a more complete fashion
- prevent the stab-in-the-dark approach of closed questioning
- allow the doctor time and space to listen and think and not just ask the next question
- contribute to more effective diagnostic reasoning
- help in the exploration of both the disease and illness frameworks
- set a pattern of patient participation rather than physician domination.

Encouraging the patient to tell their story in a more complete fashion. Closed questions give the doctor more control over the patient's responses but limit the possible information that can be obtained. Open questions, in contrast, encourage the patient to answer in an inclusive way that may well provide much more of the information that is being sought. By asking an open question, information about a problem can be obtained quickly and efficiently. In the above examples, more useful information about the chest pains was discovered with two open questions than with four closed questions.

Preventing the stab-in-the-dark approach of closed questioning. In the closed approach, all the responsibility rests on the interviewer. He has to consider which areas might be worth enquiring about and then frame appropriate questions. Clearly, the information obtained will only relate to those very areas that the doctor himself thinks are likely to be relevant and he may well forget to ask about key areas of importance. Each question is like a stab in the dark, potentially a very inefficient process. In the open method, the patient can mention areas that the interviewer might not have considered – in the above example of closed questioning, the doctor may not have thought to ask about alcohol and would have missed an important clue. This does not decry the value of closed questioning later on in the interview process. Closed questions are essential to clarify points or screen for areas not yet mentioned, but this is achieved more efficiently after a wider view of the problem has first been discovered.

Allowing the doctor time and space to listen and think and not just ask the next question. In the closed method the doctor has to follow each closed question with another. Instead of listening and thinking about the patient's replies, he is formulating the next question to keep the flow of the interview going which in turn stops him from hearing important information. The open method allows the doctor time to consider replies more carefully and pick up cues as they emerge.

Contributing to more effective diagnostic reasoning. Unless doctors use open-questioning methods at the beginning of their information gathering, it is all too easy to restrict diagnostic reasoning to an over-narrow field of enquiry. We know that doctors start the process of problem solving very early on in the consultation. They quickly attempt to match the initial information presented by the patient to their underlying knowledge of individual diseases and to organizational frameworks that they have previously developed to aid problem solving. They then direct their further questioning to prove or disprove their initial thoughts (Kassirer and Gorry 1978; Barrows and Tamblyn 1981; Gick 1986; Mandin *et al.* 1997). Open methods allow doctors more time to generate their problem-solving approach and provide them with more information on which to base their theories and hypotheses. Closed questioning, in contrast, quickly leads to the exploration of one particular avenue which may well prove inappropriate and lead inexorably to a dead-end. The doctor may have to start again and generate a different problem-solving strategy: inefficient and inaccurate information gathering ensues. In our examples above, listening to the patient's story with the use of open questions has allowed the doctor to avoid the trap of early questioning about the possibility of ischaemic heart disease and has enabled the expression of further symptoms and concerns that will help to form a more accurate working hypothesis.

Helping in the exploration of both the disease and illness frameworks. Closed questions, as explained above, are not an efficient initial method of exploring the disease aspects of a problem. They are even less helpful in discovering the illness framework. Because closed questions by their nature follow the doctor's agenda, they will tend to concentrate on the clinical aspects of the problem and omit the patient's perspective. Open questions in contrast encourage patients to talk about their illness from their unique point of view, to tell their story in their own way using their own vocabulary. Patients can choose what is important from their own perspective and the doctor can understand the patient's personal experience of their illness.

Setting a pattern of patient participation rather than physician domination. As we discussed in Chapter 2, 94% of all interruptions conclude with the doctor obtaining the floor (Beckman and Frankel 1984). The early pursuit of one problem by closed questioning shifts the whole emphasis from a patient-centred to a physician-centred format and, once this is done, the patient tends to remain in a more passive role. Once you begin closed questioning, patients will often not volunteer anything that is not explicitly asked – most patients defer to your lead. In contrast, open questions allow the patient to participate more actively, signal that it is appropriate to elaborate and make the doctor's willingness to listen apparent.

WHY IS IT IMPORTANT TO GRADUALLY MOVE FROM OPEN TO CLOSED QUESTIONING METHODS?

As the interview proceeds it is important for the doctor to become gradually more focused. She needs to use increasingly specific open questions and eventually move to closed questions to elicit fine details. Closed questions are necessary to investigate specific areas if they do not emerge from the patient's account, to analyse a symptom in detail and to take a functional enquiry (though even this can begin openly, e.g. 'Tell me about any problems with your skin ...').

Later in this chapter we explore how to move from open to closed questioning with the use of clear and explanatory transitional statements and see how summary and signposting can help overcome the perceived loss of control and potentially more disordered information gathering inherent in the use of open questioning. In Chapter 4 we will also look at the importance of accompanying non-verbal communication to the success of question-asking and see how even closed questions asked in a facilitating manner can encourage the patient to tell more of their story; good non-verbal communication can turn closed questions into open ones.

WHAT IS THE EVIDENCE FOR THE VALUE OF OPEN AND CLOSED QUESTIONING METHODS?

Roter and Hall (1987) investigated the association between primary care physicians' interviewing styles and the medical information that they obtained during consultations with simulated patients. They found that physicians on average elicited only 50% of the medical information considered important by expert consensus, with a worrying range of 9–85%! They found that the amount of information elicited was related to the use of both appropriate open and closed questions. However, open questions prompted the revelation of substantially more relevant information than closed questions.

Stiles *et al.* (1979) showed that patients at a hospital-based, medical, walk-in clinic were more satisfied with the information-gathering phase of the interview if they were allowed to express themselves in their own words rather than provide yes/no or one-word answers to closed questions.

Goldberg *et al.* (1983) investigated the ability of family practice residents in the USA to detect emotional and psychiatric problems in their patients. They looked at which aspects of residents' interview styles determined their ability to detect psychiatric disorders. Two of the skills that they found to be related to the accuracy of the residents' assessments were the open-to-closed cone and open directive rather than closed questions.

Maguire *et al.* (1996) have shown that cancer patients disclose more of their significant concerns if their doctors use open rather than leading questions.

Further evidence of the relative value of open and closed questioning comes from the detailed studies of Cox *et al.* (1981*a,b*; Rutter and Cox 1981; Cox 1989). They studied interviews with parents of children referred to a child psychiatric clinic. In the first phase of their study, they observed the interviews of trainee psychiatrists in order to determine the effects that certain interview behaviours had both on the gathering of factual information and on the expression of emotions and feelings. Their research showed:

- the ratio of open to closed questions was significantly correlated to parents' talkativeness and contributions, and the more talkative the parents, the more likely they were to bring up problems spontaneously
- the amount of talk by the interviewer, the number of topics raised by the interviewer and the number of floor-holdings were negatively correlated with parents' amount of talk and duration of utterances
- open questioning and longer utterances, encouraged by the interviewer talking less, facilitated both the expression of emotions and the gathering of sensitive data.

In the second phase of their study, experienced psychiatrists were trained to use different styles of interviewing to demonstrate that the findings from the first arm of the study could be reproduced experimentally. They were able to reproduce the findings above and also showed:

- if mothers were encouraged to express their concerns freely, they mentioned most but not quite all of the key issues without the need for closed questioning. Many of the items not raised turned out to be normal or unremarkable. In less probing styles, i.e. more open, patients mentioned more symptoms or problems that had not been previously raised or considered by the interviewer while in more probing styles, symptoms thought to be relevant by the interviewer were slightly less likely to be missed.

Their conclusion was 'that it is desirable to begin clinical diagnostic interviews with a lengthy period with little in the way of detailed probing and in which informants are allowed to express their concerns in their own way'.

Cox *et al.*'s research has also shown the value of closed questioning:

- the number of topics raised by the interviewer directly was significantly associated with a larger number of symptoms being discovered to be definitely absent, which can be very important information
- more information was obtained when interviewers used more specific requests for detailed information and more specific detailed probes per topic.

Their conclusion here was that 'if psychiatrists are to obtain sufficient detail about family problems and child symptoms for them to make an adequate formulation on which to base treatment plans, there must be some systematic and detailed probing and questioning'.

The skills of problem exploration

We have now seen the importance of employing the open-to-closed cone in information gathering. The value of starting the interview from the patient's perspective, giving the patient the floor and then gradually moving on to more specific questions cannot be over-emphasized. But what skills are available to help us put this plan into practice and explore a problem in depth?

We now explore the following framework for problem exploration:

- starting the patient off – open questioning techniques and the patient's narrative
- attentive listening
- facilitative response
- further open questions
- clarification of the patient's story
- internal summary
- more focused closed questioning including:
  - the analysis of each symptom
  - the functional enquiry related to this part of the history.

STARTING THE PATIENT OFF – OPEN QUESTIONING TECHNIQUES AND THE PATIENT'S NARRATIVE

Listening is just as important in information gathering as it is at the beginning of the consultation. But before you can start to listen, how do you set the patient off in the right direction, how do you ask the patient to give you further information about each problem?

From the discussion above, it is clear that open rather than closed methods at the beginning of problem exploration will pay dividends:

'Tell me about your headaches'

will be far more advantageous than:

'You mentioned headaches, where exactly are they?'

One particularly useful method of gathering information in an initially open way is the 'patient's narrative', encouraging the patient to tell the story of their problem from when it first started up to the present in their own words:

'Tell me all about it from the beginning.'

This is a natural way to find out about the patient's experience and to gather all the information that you need in an orderly fashion. It allows the patient to tell their story to you in much the same way as they would to a friend – people will usually have discussed their problem with several people before they come to see the doctor (Stimson and Webb 1975).

This method offers all the advantages of open questioning while providing the patient with a simple method of telling their story chronologically. It is an excellent way to understand the patient's perspective and helps prevent Mischler's 'two parallel monologues' in which patient and doctor talk at cross purposes in different languages (Mischler 1984). The role of the doctor is to listen carefully and, if necessary, to guide the patient through their story-telling, possibly seeking brief clarification but quickly returning to 'then what happened?'. The device of the patient's narrative allows the doctor to make some interruptions without necessarily taking the floor from the patient; he can return control to the patient by asking him to continue his story. However, it should be done sparingly since once the doctor has interrupted it is all too easy for him to continue in control with closed questions and forget to re-establish the patient's narrative.

ATTENTIVE LISTENING

Then, as the patient tells their story, the role of the doctor is to listen. We have already discussed the importance of attentive listening in depth in Chapter 2 when we looked at the beginning of the interview. As we have seen, attentive listening is a highly skilled process, requiring a combination of facilitative responses, wait time and picking up cues.

If we look again at the advantages of attentive listening, we can see how many features are shared with the advantages of open questions mentioned earlier in this chapter. This similarity is because attentive listening is a direct consequence of the use of open questions; it is almost impossible to employ active listening and closed questioning together.

FACILITATIVE RESPONSE

As well as listening, it is important to actively encourage patients to continue their story-telling. Closed questioning is so predominant that patients may well initially respond even to excellent open questions with only a word or two unless they are encouraged to continue. Any behaviour that has the effect of inviting patients to say more about the area that they are already discussing is a facilitative response. When we began our discussion of facilitative responses in Chapter 2, we looked at the research evidence showing that certain skills such as echoing or repetition could be counter-productive when used too early in the interview. At the beginning of the interview, our objective is to obtain as wide a view as possible of the patient's whole agenda before exploring any one problem in detail. Now let us turn our attention to the use of facilitative responses in the information-gathering phase. What are the skills that are useful here when we are trying to encourage patients to talk about each of their problems in greater depth?

The facilitative response involves both verbal and non-verbal communication skills. In this chapter we focus primarily on verbal communication and discuss selected non-verbal skills. We explore non-verbal communication in greater depth in Chapter 4.

The following skills can be used to facilitate the patient to say more about a topic, indicating simultaneously that you are interested in what they are saying and that you are keen for them to continue:

- encouragement
- silence
- repetition (echoing)
- paraphrasing.

Encouragement

Along with non-verbal head nods and the use of facial expression, doctors practising attentive listening use frequent verbal encouragers which signal the patient to continue their story. This is often achieved very efficiently with minimal or no interruption and yet provides the patient with the necessary confidence to keep going. Such neutral facilitative comments include *'uh-huh'*, *'go on'*, *'yes'*, *'um'*, *'I see'* – we all have our own particular favourites.

Use of silence

Most verbal facilitation is ineffective unless immediately followed by attentive silence. In Chapter 2, we discussed the work of Rowe (1986) on wait time and how the use of brief silence or pause can very easily and naturally facilitate the patient to contribute more. Longer periods of silence are also appropriate if the patient is having difficulty in expressing themselves or if it seems that the patient is about to be overwhelmed by emotion. The aim of providing a longer pause is to encourage the patient to express out loud the thoughts or feelings that are occurring inside their head. There is a delicate balance here between comfortable and uncomfortable silence, between encouraging communication and interfering with it by creating uncertainty and anxiety: the doctor must attend carefully to accompanying non-verbal behaviour. However, remember that anxiety is more often felt by the clinician than the patient; patients usually tolerate silence better than doctors!

If the clinician does feel that a silence is producing anxiety or the patient eventually needs further encouragement to speak, particular attention must be given to how the silence is broken. For instance,

'Can you bear to tell me what you are thinking?'

acts to allow the patient to stay with their thoughts and further facilitates the process – as does repetition of the patient's last words, as we will see below.

Repetition or echoing

Repeating the last few words that the patient has said encourages the patient to keep talking. Doctors often worry that this 'echoing' will sound unnatural but again it is remarkably well accepted by patients. Note how repetition encourages the patient to continue with their last phrase and is therefore slightly more directive than encouragement or silence. This explains Beckman and Frankel's (1984) work, discussed in Chapter 2, which showed that echoing could act as a possible interrupter at the beginning of the interview by forcing the patient down a specific path before the doctor had discovered the full spectrum of concerns.

Following through the example we used earlier, we can see the above skills in action:

Doctor: *'Tell me about the chest pain that you have been having.'* (open question)
Patient: *'Well, it's been building up over the last few weeks. I've always had a little indigestion but not as bad as this. I get this sharp pain right here* (pointing to sternum) *and then I belch a lot and get a really horrible acid taste in my mouth. Its much worse if I've had a drink or two and I'm not getting much sleep.'*
Doctor: *'Yes, go on'* (encouragement)
Patient: *'Well, I was wondering if it was brought on by the pills I've been taking for my joints – they've been much worse and I got some ibuprofen from the drug-store. I need to keep going at the moment what with John and all.'*
Doctor: (silence – accompanied by eye contact, slight head nod)
Patient: *'He's really going downhill, doctor and I don't know how I'm going to cope at home if he gets any worse.'*
Doctor: *'How you're going to cope?'* (repetition)
Patient: *'I promised him I wouldn't let him go into hospital again and now I'm not sure if I can do it.'*

Paraphrasing

Paraphrasing is restating in your own words the content or feelings behind the patient's message. It is not quite the same as checking or summarizing (see below): it is intended to sharpen rather than just confirm understanding and therefore tends to be more specific than the original message. Paraphrasing checks if your own *interpretation* of what the patient actually means is correct. Continuing our example:

Doctor: *'Are you thinking that when John gets even more ill, you won't be strong enough to nurse him at home by yourself?'* (paraphrase of content)
Patient: *'I think I'll be OK physically, but what happens if he needs me day and night – there's only me and I can't call on Mary, what with her job.'*
Doctor: *'It sounds as if you're worried that you might be letting John down.'* (paraphrase of feeling)

Paraphrasing combines elements of facilitation, summarizing and clarification. It is particularly helpful if you think that you understand but are not quite certain or you think that there might be hidden feelings behind a seemingly simple message. Paraphrasing is a very good facilitative entry point into the patient's illness framework.

WHAT IS THE THEORETICAL EVIDENCE FOR FACILITATION?

The facilitative skills enumerated above are the key skills of non-directive counselling. They have been extensively discussed by Rogers (1980), Egan (1990) and others and are widely accepted as crucial elements of any communication in which the aim is to encourage the client to talk more about their problem without undue professional direction.

There is little specific research work on each of these skills as applied to medical interviews and it is therefore difficult to provide research data to support their individual use. However, Levinson *et al.* (1997) showed that primary care physicians who used more facilitation statements (soliciting patients' opinions, checking understanding, encouraging patients to talk, paraphrasing and interpretation) were less likely to have suffered malpractice claims. This association was not found for surgeons in the same study.

Collectively, facilitation skills form a major part of the patient-centred interviewing style (Henbest and Stewart 1990*a,b*) which, as we discuss in the next section, has been demonstrated to favourably affect many measurable parameters of communication. Patient-centredness in these studies was scored by a combination of open-ended questions, facilitative expressions and specific requests for patients' expectations, thoughts and feelings in response to patients' comments.

FURTHER OPEN QUESTIONS

As the interview proceeds, the doctor may need to become more directive, guiding the patient to elaborate further on specific areas that have surfaced as they tell their story. He does this by employing more direct verbal encouragement in the form of open statements and questions:

- *'Tell me more about the pain.'*
- *'You mentioned breathlessness, tell me about that.'*
- *'Did you notice anything else while all this was going on?'*
- *'And what did you do then?'*

CLARIFICATION OF THE PATIENT'S STORY

Obtaining clarification of statements which are vague or need further amplification is a vital information-gathering skill. After an initial response to an open-ended question, the doctor may need to prompt the patient for more precision, clarity or completeness. Often, patients' statements can have two possible meanings; it is important to ascertain which one is intended.

Clarifying is often open in nature:

'Could you explain what you mean by light-headed?'

but may also be closed:

'When you say dizzy, do you mean that the room seems to actually spin around?'.

If the patient does not provide dates for important events in their history, ask for them. Check that you understand the sequence of events correctly if you are uncertain. And to improve accuracy, learn to timeframe your own questions. Compare:

'Have you experienced depression?' (undated)
'Have you ever experienced depression?'
'Have you experienced depression in the last two weeks since you hit your head?'

Too often we ask the first when we mean the third. When patients answer *'occasionally'*, which question were they answering?

INTERNAL SUMMARY

Summarizing is the deliberate step of making an explicit verbal summary to the patient of the information gathered so far and is one of the most important of all information-gathering skills. Used periodically throughout the interview, summarizing is a key method of ensuring accuracy in the consultation. It allows the patient to confirm that you have understood what they have said or to correct your misinterpretation and also acts as an excellent facilitative opening by inviting and allowing the patient to go further in explaining their problems and thoughts.

Doctor: *'Can I just see if I've got this right? You've had indigestion before, but for the last few weeks you've had increasing problems with a sharp pain at the front of your chest, accompanied by wind and acid. It's stopping you from sleeping, it's made worse by drink and you were wondering if the painkillers were to blame. Is that right?'* (Pause ...)
Patient: *'Yes, and I can't afford to be ill now with John being so sick. I don't know how I'm going to cope.'*

Summarizing plays a vital role in two separate but related aspects of information gathering, *exploring patient's problems* and *structuring the consultation*. We explore both of these roles in detail later in this chapter.

MORE FOCUSED CLOSED QUESTIONING

As the exploration of the problem progresses, the emphasis shifts from the patient's perspective to the doctor's. There are important facets of the medical history that may well not have emerged from the patient's account and the gradual movement from open to closed questioning enables the practitioner to ensure that these areas are explored. For example, a patient with non-organic-sounding chest pain might not overtly mention stress as possibly contributing to their symptoms. After careful listening and the judicial use of open questions, the doctor might ask the specific closed question:

'Are you under a lot of stress at the moment?'
'Well, my daughter's marriage has been breaking up recently.'

Be careful that your closed questioning is not too focused. It is easy to ask the patient an inappropriate closed question: we think ahead too quickly, think of a possible answer to a question we have posed to ourselves and then test our own premature hypothesis. Instead, ask the question that was in your mind right from the start! A good example of this would be where the doctor above wonders if his patient is under any stresses at the moment. Instead of asking a general question such as *'Are there any stresses in your life at the moment?'*, he thinks ahead and wonders if she is having problems at home and asks *'Are things OK with your husband at present?'*. The patient says 'fine' and the doctor moves on without an answer to his original question.

The analysis of each symptom
As the interview shifts to a more disease-orientated focus, the doctor needs to ensure that valuable diagnostic data are not omitted. We would like to emphasize at this point the importance of a thorough analysis of each symptom, an approach that the traditional methodology of history taking has always stressed. Box 3.2 contains two examples of

---

Box 3.2   Content required to investigate a symptom

WWQQAA plus B

1 Where – the location and radiation of a symptom
2 When – when it began, fluctuation over time, duration
3 Quality – what it feels like
4 Quantity – intensity, extent, degree of disability
5 Aggravating and alleviating factors
6 Associated manifestations – other symptoms
7 Beliefs – the patient's beliefs about the symptoms

Macleod's clinical examination (Macleod 1964)

1 Site
2 Radiation
3 Character
4 Severity
5 Duration
6 Frequency and periodicity
7 Special times of occurrence
8 Aggravating factors
9 Relieving factors
10 Associated phenomena

aides-mémoire that list the content required to investigate a symptom and thereby help us to be systematic in our approach.

Again, these more directive questions can be open at first and then increasingly closed if necessary:

'Can you describe what the pain felt like?'
'Was it a sharp pain?'

The functional enquiry
A further element that requires closed questioning is the functional enquiry or systems review appropriate to the particular part of the medical history being explored. As we have seen, important information is lost if a systematic approach to the exclusion of associated symptoms is not employed. Although it may only discover which symptoms are definitely absent, this is still highly useful diagnostic information that cannot otherwise be assumed.

Further skills in problem exploration

Two other skills are also valuable in problem exploration. As they feature prominently in other chapters of the book, we discuss them only briefly here:

1 *Language*. The use of concise, easily understood questions and comments, without jargon, is important throughout the interview. We concentrate on this aspect of communication when we explore explanation and planning in Chapter 5.
2 *Sharing your thoughts*. Sharing why you are asking questions is another excellent way of phrasing questions and encouraging the patient to be inclusive in their answer. For example:

'Sometimes, chest pains can be brought on by stress – I was wondering if you felt that might be true for you, whether you were under a lot of stress at present?'

This is ostensibly a closed question but the fact that the patient can understand the reasoning behind your request allows her to answer and then elaborate. The more direct 'Are you under a lot of stress at present?' is far more likely to produce a one-word response. We discuss the issue of sharing your thoughts with the patient further in Chapter 4.

SECTION 2: UNDERSTANDING THE PATIENT'S PERSPECTIVE

What is the evidence to support the value of exploring the patient's perspective of their illness?

Earlier in this chapter, we looked in detail at the disease–illness model and the importance of exploring both the doctor's and the patient's frameworks in the consultation. We would now like to examine the research evidence that validates the importance of understanding the patient's perspective of their illness.

The patient's illness framework includes:

• ideas or beliefs (about the causation or effect of the illness, about health and what influences or contributes to it)

- concerns (worries about what symptoms might mean)
- expectations (hopes of how the doctor might help)
- thoughts and feelings (emotions and thoughts that the illness induces)
- effects on life (the effect the illness has on day-to-day living).

ANTHROPOLOGICAL AND CROSS-CULTURAL STUDIES

Many of the concepts that helped to formulate the disease–illness model came originally from anthropological and cross-cultural studies. Kleinman *et al.*'s (1978) seminal review paper brought together the lessons from qualitative anthropological research and explained how the results of this work can be applied to everyday medical interviews.

The authors explore how patients' explanatory frameworks of their illness are culturally shaped. Our social, cultural and spiritual beliefs about health and illness influence our perception of our symptoms, expectations about our illness and our help-seeking behaviour (from families, friends and professionals). Illness behaviour is governed by cultural rules with marked cross-cultural variations in how disorders are both defined by society and dealt with by the individual. These differences also exist within a given culture across class and family boundaries.

It is not only patients' beliefs that are culturally determined but doctors' beliefs too! Even within modern Western medical practice itself, there are large cultural differences that determine what is perceived as 'clinical reality'. We have all noticed marked differences in explanations and treatment that physicians from other parts of the world have given our patients during holidays abroad. The biomedical viewpoint is also 'culture specific and value laden' rather than, as we so often think, 'objective'.

Kleinman *et al.* (1978) quote examples of the wide range of explanatory frameworks of illness in ethnic minorities living in the USA. For instance, Chinese and Guatemalan patients' understanding of illness differs markedly from the biomedical perspective of their American-trained doctors. Often, cultural minorities will not respond to illness in the way expected by their professional advisors. In Chinese cultural settings, for example, mental illness is highly stigmatized and minor psychiatric disorders are commonly manifested by somatization.

The authors then proceed to explore the relevance of differences between the explanatory models of doctor and patient within a single culture. In their model, multicultural interviews simply represent an extreme example of all medical encounters. In all patient–doctor inter-actions, there is potential for differences in explanatory models which can inhibit effective communication.

In a study of health beliefs related to culture in a multicultural urban setting Chugh *et al.* (1994) showed clearly that beliefs within a cultural group are often as diverse as beliefs between cultural groups. Understanding the diversity of health beliefs related to culture is important but it is still essential to discover the health beliefs of each individual patient.

Kleinman *et al.* (1978) recommend that doctors should not only elicit their patient's explanatory model but also openly compare and discuss the patient's and doctor's conflicting ideas. This they see as an essential step to improving compliance with medical advice which is likely to be poor if the doctor has not explained his recommendations in relation to his patient's beliefs and if the doctor's advice does not seem to help with the problem as the patient sees it. This is the stage labelled 'integration' in the disease–illness model (see Fig. 3.1). Only by discovering the patient's illness framework can we explain and plan in terms the patient can understand and accept. The patient's ideas and beliefs, concerns and expectations need to be built into our explanation of the disease process so that we cover the questions that are most important from the patient's perspective and together reach some degree of common ground. It is important to get to a position where our explanations and recommendations make sense in the patient's world. Therefore, exploring the patient's beliefs involves a three-stage process:

1 **identification** – discover and listen to the patient's ideas, concerns and expectations
2 **acceptance** – acknowledge the patient's views and their right to hold them, without necessarily agreeing with them
3 **explanation** – explain your understanding of the problem in relation to the patient's understanding and reach mutually understood common ground.

We discuss acceptance in greater depth in Chapter 4 and explore this three-stage model further in Chapter 5 when we look at Tuckett *et al.*'s (1985) work on the influence that eliciting the patient's explanatory framework has on the patient's recall and understanding of our explanations.

Wright *et al.* (1996) add further depth to our understanding of the patient's perspective. In their recent book on beliefs in health care, they substantiate the point that what patients believe about their illness – treatment, aetiology, prognosis, the role of health in their lives, relationships between spirituality and health – has more influence on how they cope with illness than any other factor. Their book also explores the positive role clinicians can play in understanding, building on and influencing those beliefs.

OUTCOME STUDIES

What evidence do we have that eliciting patients' own perspectives about their illness actually affects disease outcome?

The Headache Study Group of the University of Western Ontario (1986) performed a one-year prospective study of 272 patients presenting to family physicians with a new complaint of headache. The purpose of the study was to describe the natural history of headache in primary care and to assess the importance of possible variables to the successful resolution of the headaches after one year. The group looked at many different variables including physician diagnosis, organic or non-organic diagnosis, the presence of certain symptoms, treatment, investigation, referral, age, sex and the presence of psychosocial problems. While treatment, investigation and referral made no impact on symptom resolution at a year, the most important of all the possible variables was the patient's perception that they had been able to fully discuss their headaches and the problems surrounding them at the first visit (3.4 times more likely to have full resolution). An organic diagnosis (3.2) and lack of visual symptoms (2.2) were the other two most important factors. This paper clearly demonstrates the importance of doctor–patient communication to the outcome of chronic headache.

Orth *et al.* (1987) showed that reduction of blood pressure was significantly greater in hypertensive patients who, during visits to the doctor, were allowed to express their health concerns in their own words without interruption, as opposed to answering yes/no questions.

Brody and Miller (1986) looked at recovery from upper respiratory infections in patients attending a hospital walk-in clinic. Whereas symptom type and severity, initial level of health concern, findings on examination, culture result and therapy appeared to be unrelated to speed of recovery, recovery was related to reduction in concerns after the visit (particularly about the seriousness of the problem and its consequences for the future) and to patient satisfaction with the helpfulness of time spent discussing concerns.

Roter *et al.* (1995) showed in a randomized controlled trial that training physicians in primary care in 'problem-defining and emotion-handling skills' (which included many of the skills of exploring the illness framework) not only improved the detection and management of psychosocial problems but also led to a reduction in patients' emotional distress for as long as six months.

SATISFACTION AND COMPLIANCE STUDIES

Many studies document the relationship between a patient-centred approach and patient satisfaction and compliance. Korsch *et al.* (1968) and Frances *et al.* (1969), in their seminal study of 800 visits to a paediatric walk-in out-patients in Los Angeles, were among the first researchers to tackle the doctor–patient interaction using rigorous methods. Satisfaction and compliance with the consultation were shown to be reduced if doctors demonstrated:

• lack of warmth and friendliness
• failure to take parents' concerns and expectations into account
• use of jargon
• lack of clear explanations of diagnosis and causation.

Korsch *et al.* showed that mothers' expectations were often not elicited by the paediatrician and that only 24% of mothers' main worries were mentioned. Lack of heed of mothers' expressed worry or expectation led mothers to 'click off' from the interview and give little further information. On the other hand, when the needs that mothers perceived to be urgent were met, mothers appeared attentive and amenable to the doctors' ideas and plans. The highest incidence of dissatisfaction on follow-up occurred in those visits where neither expectations or main concern received attention. No further time was taken when expectations were discovered.

Joos *et al.* (1993) and Kravitz *et al.* (1994) have also shown, both in patients with chronic medical conditions and in those attending internal medicine out-patients, that patients were significantly more satisfied if their prior expectations of help were fulfilled in the interview. However, many patients' desires for further information about their disease or medication or for help with emotional and family problems remained unmet.

Eisenthal and Lazare, in a series of classic studies on the 'customer approach' to patients in a psychiatric walk-in clinic (Lazare *et al.* 1975; Eisenthal and Lazare 1976; Eisenthal *et al.* 1979; 1990), extensively studied patients' expectations by looking specifically at 'how the patient hoped the doctor might help them' as well as at their presenting symptoms. They clearly demonstrated that patients' expectations are often not obvious from the chief complaint, that clinicians need to make a specific enquiry to discover their patients' expectations and that doctors do not routinely ask for patients' expectations. Their research showed that if physicians did ask for patients' expectations, patients were more likely to feel satisfied and helped and also to adhere to a negotiated plan. Most importantly, their research clearly demonstrated that this increased satisfaction was apparent regardless of whether or not the request was granted. This is a very significant finding: in Korsch's (1968) and Joos' (1993) work, the positive relationship between expectations and satisfaction related to patients' expectations being fulfilled rather than just elicited. This is perhaps not surprising: if patients get what they wanted, they feel happier. But what if expectations are elicited and discussed but not eventually granted? Is the fact that the expectation is still unmet still a cause for dissatisfaction or is the process of discovery and negotiation helpful in itself?

Eisenthal and Lazare (1976) have shown that eliciting and addressing the expectation is indeed of value in itself, that a negotiated treatment plan based on an understanding of the patient's expectations is helpful. In other words, it is not finding out whether the patient wants antibiotics for their cough and going along with their wishes that is important but finding out patients' expectations and explaining your position in relation to their views. This fits in with the three-stage plan of exploring beliefs outlined above. Basing our negotiation on an open understanding of our respective positions and reaching mutually understood common ground is the final aim.

Little *et al.* (1997), in an open randomized trial of the management of sore throat in primary care, showed that satisfaction with the consultation predicted the duration of illness and was strongly related to how well the doctor dealt with patient concerns.

Stewart (1984) audio-taped 140 consultations in primary care and analysed physician behaviour to determine how 'patient-centred' they were in terms of seeking the patient's views and facilitating the patient's self-expression and asking of questions. Patients were then interviewed in their homes ten days later. She demonstrated that a high frequency of patient-centred behaviour was related to higher compliance and satisfaction.

Henbest and Stewart (1990*a,b*) took this work further by developing a specific tool for measuring the degree to which physicians allowed the patient to express their feelings, thoughts and expectations. Patient-centredness in these studies was scored by a combination of open-ended questions, facilitative expressions and specific requests for patients' expectations, thoughts and feelings. Patient-centredness was found to be significantly related to the doctor ascertaining the patient's reasons for coming and with resolution of the patient's concerns.

Arborelius and Bremberg (1992) showed in a study in general practice that successful consultations, where both doctor and patient rated the interview positively, were characterized by increased efforts being made to establish the patient's ideas and concerns and with more time being spent on the tasks of shared understanding and involving the patient in their own management.

UNDERSTANDING AND RECALL STUDIES

Tuckett *et al.*'s (1985) research on information giving, which we explore more fully in Chapter 5, demonstrates the great importance of eliciting patients' beliefs and views of their illness in enabling patients to understand and recall information provided by the doctor. Yet, their research efforts were hampered by the very few examples that they were able to find at all of doctors asking patients to volunteer their ideas or even of doctors asking the patient to elaborate on their ideas if they were spontaneously brought up. Doctors often evaded their patients' ideas and positively inhibited their expression; this behaviour led to a considerably increased likelihood of failure of understanding and recall.

Doctor understanding is also enhanced by patient-centred interviewing. Peppiatt (1992) showed in a study of 1000 interviews undertaken by one family physician that 77% of patients either spontaneously offered or responded to requests to express a cause for their condition and that 20% of patients' ideas of causation helped the doctor decide on a cause, with 9% enabling the doctor to actually make a diagnosis.

ARE PATIENT-CENTRED INTERVIEWS LONGER?

Stewart (1985) looked at 133 interviews in primary care and compared their 'patient-centredness' score with the length of the consultation. Low scores for patient-centredness produced interviews of on average 7.8 minutes, intermediate scores 10.9 minutes and high scores 8.5 minutes. Her conclusion was that doctors can expect to take longer while they learn the skills. But doctors who have *mastered* the patient-centred approach took little extra time compared with doctors not employing these techniques.

Roter *et al.* (1995) also found no increase in the length of interviews in primary care following training in the skills of 'problem defining and emotion handling'.

Levinson and Roter (1995) showed that primary care physicians with more positive attitudes to psychosocial aspects of patient care used more appropriate communication skills and as a consequence their patients had more psychosocial discussions and were more involved as partners in their own care. Yet these same physicians did not have longer interviews than colleagues with less positive attitudes.

How to discover the patient's perspective

There are two alternative ways of exploring the patient's illness framework as the interview proceeds. The first is by directly asking for the patient's ideas, concerns, expectations and feelings; the second is by picking up cues provided by the patient during the course of the consultation. Maguire *et al.* (1996) have demonstrated the value of both of these techniques. Cancer patients disclosed more of their significant concerns and feelings if doctors asked them questions about psychological aspects of their care (*'How has that made you feel?'*) rather than concentrating solely on physical aspects of their disease. They also disclosed more concerns if doctors specifically clarified psychological cues that arose (*'You say that you have been worrying …'*). As predicted, the use of open questions, summarizing and empathic statements also promoted disclosure of concerns.

PICKING UP AND CHECKING OUT CUES

Patients are keen to disclose their own thoughts and feelings. In Tuckett *et al.*'s (1985) research, 26% of patients spontaneously offered an explanation of their symptoms to the doctor. However, when patients did express their views, only 7% of doctors actively encouraged their patients to elaborate, 13% listened passively and 81% made no effort to listen or deliberately interrupted. Half of patients' views were expressed covertly rather than overtly with overt cues being picked up far more readily than covert cues. The conclusion here is that many patients provide cues which doctors unfortunately ignore!

We have already described the work of Cox *et al.* (1981a,b; Rutter and Cox 1981; Cox 1989) who showed that open questioning and attentive listening facilitated both the expression of emotions and the gathering of sensitive data with a high emotional significance. If the doctor establishes an atmosphere of interest and openness, many of the patient's feelings and thoughts will appear as cues in the attentive listening stage. It can then be a relatively easy and natural process to pick up and explore these cues further. This often feels more comfortable for both patient and doctor than the asking of direct, unprompted questions.

It should be emphasized that cues do not only appear as verbal comments. Non-verbal cues in body language, speech, facial expression and affect are also highly significant. To ensure accurate interpretation of such non-verbal behaviour, it is important to observe carefully and then sensitively verify your perceptions with the patient.

But why do doctors repeatedly fail to pick up patients' cues? Perhaps it is due in part to issues of control. Doctors have traditionally controlled the interview via closed questions which limit patients' contributions and render them more passive. When we pick up patient cues, perhaps we feel that we are being taken off our pre-planned flightpath and are uncertain of where we might be led; we start to feel out of control. Paradoxically, cues are usually a shortcut to important areas requiring attention. We may also fail to pick up cues to the illness framework because we are preferentially listening for cues about disease. If the patient says *'It's been difficult at home and I've been getting a lot more pains lately'*, it is so easy to preferentially pick up the disease rather than the illness cue and say *'Tell me about the pains'* without returning to *'You mentioned things have been difficult at home ...'*. Box 3.3 contains examples of ways to pick up verbal and non-verbal cues.

Box 3.3   Ways to pick up verbal and non-verbal cues

Repetition of cues

- 'upset ...?'
- 'something could be done ...?'

Picking up and checking out verbal cues

- 'You said that you were worried that the pain might be something serious; what theories did you have yourself about what it might be?'
- 'You mentioned that your mother had rheumatoid arthritis; did you think that's what might be happening to you?'

Picking up and checking out non-verbal cues

- 'I sense that you're not quite happy with the explanations you've been given in the past. Is that right?'
- 'Am I right in thinking you're quite upset about your daughter's illness?'

ASKING SPECIFICALLY ABOUT THE PATIENT'S ILLNESS PERSPECTIVE

Although picking up patient cues might be easier, asking specifically about the illness perspective is still a very necessary task. Yet in Tuckett's (1985) work, only 6% of doctors asked patients directly for their own thoughts about their illness. Direct questions need careful timing, with good signposting of intent and attention to detail in wording. Bass and Cohen (1982) showed that when parents in a paediatric practice were asked *'What worries you about this problem?'*, the majority of parents responded with *'I'm not worried'* whereas the phrase

'What concerns you about the problem?' produced previously unrecognized concerns in more than a third of parents.

Different phrasing is required to ask questions about patients' ideas, concerns or expectations (Box 3.4).

Box 3.4 Examples of phrasing when asking about patients' ideas, concerns or expectations

---

Ideas (beliefs)

- 'Tell me about what you think is causing it.'
- 'What do you think might be happening?'
- 'Have you any ideas about it yourself?'
- 'Do you have any clues; any theories?'
- 'You've obviously given this some thought, it would help me to know what you were thinking it might be.'

Concerns

- 'What are you concerned that it might be?'
- 'Is there anything particular or specific that you were concerned about?'
- 'What was the worst thing you were thinking it might be?'
- 'In your darkest moments ...'

Expectations

- 'What were you hoping we might be able to do for this?'
- 'What do you think might be the best plan of action?'
- 'How might I best help you with this?'
- 'You've obviously given this some thought, what were you thinking would be the best way of tackling this?'

FEELINGS

Many doctors find entering the realm of patients' feelings particularly difficult. It does not fit naturally with the objective approach of the traditional clinical method and is something which at medical school we were often taught to avoid. Impassive objectivity can be appealing; feelings are often difficult to handle and may be painful to the doctor as well as the patient. Doctors are frightened of 'opening a Pandora's box' of their patients' emotions and feelings. In comparison, it is the area that other professionals such as counsellors and therapists are most encouraged to explore! It is therefore particularly important to become aware of and practise the skills involved in discovering and responding to patients' feelings (Box 3.5).

Box 3.5   Skills involved in discovering and responding to patients' feelings

---

Picking up and checking out verbal cues

- 'You said you felt miserable, could you tell me more about how you've been feeling?'

Repetition of verbal cues

- 'angry ...?'

Picking up and reflecting non-verbal cues

- 'I sense that you're very tense; would it help to talk about it?' or 'You sound sad when you talk about John.'

Direct questions

- 'How did that leave you feeling?'

Using acceptance, empathy, concern and understanding to signal to the patient that you are interested in their feelings (see Chapter 4)

- 'I can see that must have been hard for you.'

Early use of feelings questions to establish your interest in the subject

Asking for particular examples

- 'Can you remember a time when you felt like that? What actually happened?'

Asking permission to enter the feelings realm

- 'Could you bear to tell me just how you have been feeling?'

How to end the discussion of feelings and not sink into a downward spiral with the patient

- 'Thank you for telling me how you have been feeling. It helps me to understand the situation much better. Do you think you've told me enough about how you are feeling to help me understand things?' or 'I think I understand now a little of what you have been feeling. Let's look at the practical things that we can do together to help.'

EFFECT ON LIFE

An open question about how the symptoms or illness are affecting the patient's life is an excellent entry into the patient's perspective of the problem and, in particular, often leads the patient to talk openly about their thoughts and feelings.

SECTION 3: PROVIDING STRUCTURE TO THE CONSULTATION

Internal summary

As we pointed out earlier in this chapter, summarizing is one of the most important of all information-gathering skills. It plays a vital role in two separate but related aspects of information gathering, *exploring patients' problems* and *structuring the consultation*.

WHAT IS SUMMARIZING?

Summarizing is the deliberate step of making an explicit verbal summary to the patient of the information gathered so far. There are two kinds of summary: *internal summary* which focuses on a specific part of the interview and *end summary* which concisely pulls together the entire interview. Used periodically throughout the interview, summarizing is a key method of ensuring accuracy in the consultation.

Doctor: *'Can I just see if I've got this right? You've had indigestion before, but for the last few weeks you've had increasing problems with a sharp pain at the front of your chest, accompanied by wind and acid. It's stopping you from sleeping, it's made worse by drink and you were wondering if the painkillers were to blame. Is that right? (Pause ...)*
Patient: *'Yes, and I can't afford to be ill now with John being so sick. I don't know how I'm going to cope.'*

WHY IS INTERNAL SUMMARY A KEY SKILL IN EXPLORING THE PATIENT'S PROBLEMS?

The advantages of internal summary for the patient:

- clearly demonstrates that you have been listening
- demonstrates that you are interested and care about getting things right
- offers a collaborative approach to problem solving
- allows the patient to check your understanding and thoughts
- gives the patient an opportunity to either confirm or correct your interpretation and add in missing areas
- invites and allows the patient to go further in explaining their problems and thoughts by acting as a facilitative opening
- demonstrates the doctor's interest in the illness as well as the disease aspects of the patient's story.

The advantages of internal summary for the doctor:

- maximizes accurate information gathering by allowing you to check the accuracy of what you think the patient has said and rectify any misconceptions; promotes mutually under-stood common ground
- provides a space for you to review what you have already covered
- allows you to order your thoughts and clarify in your mind what you are not sure about and what aspect of the story you need to explore next
- allows you to separate and consider both disease and illness.

Summarizing is one of the most important information-gathering tools at our disposal and can be used frequently in the course of interviewing to great effect. It is an excellent practical test of whether you have understood the patient correctly and will make you not only more accurate in the consultation but also more far reaching in your understanding of the patient's problems. Summary followed by a pause and attentive listening is an important method of enabling the patient to continue their story without explicit direction from the doctor; it acts as a facilitative opening by inviting and allowing the patient to go further in explaining their problems and thoughts.

It is important to remember to summarize both the disease and illness aspects of the patient's story. Summarizing both is an excellent method of helping to fulfil two of our previously stated objectives for this phase of the interview:

1 exploring and understanding the patient's perspective so as to understand the meaning of the illness for the patient
2 exploring the disease framework so as to obtain an adequate 'medical' history.

Summarizing tells you whether you have 'got it right'. If you have, the patient will confirm your picture with both verbal and non-verbal signs of agreement. If, however, your understanding is inaccurate or incomplete, the patient will tell you or provide non-verbal signals of being unhappy (Neighbour 1987). Without an overt verbal summary, we inappropriately rely on conjecture and assumption that we have understood our patients correctly.

WHAT IS THE EVIDENCE FOR THE VALUE OF SUMMARIZING IN INFORMATION GATHERING?

We have only identified two research papers which validate the importance of summarizing. Cox *et al.* (1981*a*) demonstrated that checking by repetition led parents of children referred to a child psychiatric clinic to be more voluble. Maguire *et al.* (1996) showed that summarizing is one of several skills (along with the use of open questions, focusing on and clarifying psychological aspects, empathic statements and making educated guesses) that facilitates cancer patients to disclose more of their significant concerns.

Despite this lack of direct medical research, there is impressive theoretical evidence from the discipline of communication studies to underpin the value of summarizing. In Chapter 1, we described five principles that characterize effective communication. One of these principles is that *effective communication is a helical rather than a linear process – reiteration and repetition are essential.* Summary is an efficient way to build this principle into information gathering. A second and related principle is that *effective communication ensures an interaction rather than a direct transmission process.* If communication is viewed as direct transmission, the senders of messages assume that their responsibilities as communicators are fulfilled once they have formulated and sent a message. However, if communication is viewed as an interactive process, the interaction is complete only if the sender receives feedback about how the message is interpreted, whether it is understood and what impact it has on the receiver. Just imparting information or just listening is not enough: giving and receiving feedback about the impact of the message becomes crucial and the emphasis moves to the interdependence of sender and receiver in establishing mutually understood common ground (Dance and Larson 1972). Summarizing is the key skill in the information-gathering phase of the interview that enables this principle to be put into practice; it provides intentional feedback to the patient about what you think you have heard when listening to their story. As we shall see later, further skills are required in the explanation and planning phase to ensure a similar degree of interaction.

Let us look further at these critical concepts. Without feedback from the doctor, how does the patient know whether he has made himself understood? You might say that non-verbal cues are being transmitted by the doctor in attentive listening that allow the patient to know that the doctor is concentrating on and interested in his story and has understood his message. But this is an assumption. We cannot assume that exemplary listening by itself leads to correct understanding – communication is complicated and many misinterpretations are possible. The key question to ask yourself as a doctor is 'How do I know that what I have understood from the patient is an accurate representation of what they wanted to tell me?'. From the patient's perspective, the question becomes 'I know that the doctor seems to be listening but how do I know that he has understood me?'. How do both patient and doctor know that they have established mutually understood common ground?

There are many possible sources of distortion in communication as any message is sent between two parties. Consider a patient giving their story to a doctor. Possible distortion can occur at the following points:

- what the patient says might be ambiguous
- the patient may have simply forgotten to say something
- the patient may have misunderstood the doctor's question
- having already told their story to one member of the health care team, the patient may assume this new individual already knows it
- the patient may have been led off the topic and never returned to complete the unfinished comment
- the patient may have inadvertently made a verbal mistake that distorts his meaning
- the patient may give a non-verbal cue such as a laugh which suggests something unintended to the doctor
- the patient may have said exactly what he meant but distortion occurred in the circumstances of transmission of the message – a noisy printer prevents the doctor hearing fully what was said
- the doctor hears the correct message but misinterprets what was meant
- the doctor understands what was meant but makes an incorrect assumption about what lay behind the message
- the doctor may have personal biases and prejudices which affect accuracy (e.g. based on gender or race or age of the patient, the doctor's medical training, the location of the interview, previous experience with the patient).

All these distortions can lead to inaccurate history taking. The only way to be sure that the message has been formulated properly, received correctly and interpreted and understood is through feedback. In the doctor–patient interview, it is unlikely that the patient will feel confident enough to ask us to demonstrate our understanding of their story! Unless we as doctors take responsibility by giving feedback via summary as the interview proceeds, we will leave the patient uncertain as to whether they have been understood and we ourselves will be unsure that we have obtained an accurate account.

It is helpful to use a signposting statement to introduce and draw attention to your first summary; this announces what you are going to do and invites patients to think with you, to add in forgotten areas or correct your interpretation if you have got something wrong. For instance, by saying: *'Can I just check if I have understood you – let me know if I've missed something? ...'* Then the interactive process can continue: *'No, that's not quite right ...'*

WHY IS INTERNAL SUMMARY A KEY SKILL IN STRUCTURING THE CONSULTATION?

Having demonstrated the importance of internal summary in exploring the patient's problems, we now describe its second and equally vital role in structuring the consultation. Understanding how to structure a consultation via *agenda setting, summarizing* and *signposting* is a key area in communication skills teaching and learning.

Traditionally, doctors have controlled the consultation via closed questions which, as we explained earlier, keep them 'in control' at the expense of rendering the patient passive. But as we have seen, this approach can be an inefficient and inaccurate way to obtain quality information and can feel unsupportive to the patient. So if staying open and using attentive listening is so effective, why do we shy away from it? Perhaps it is because:

- it can feel like we have lost control of the consultation
- we worry that we will not need or be able to remember all that we are being told
- information flows out in a less ordered form – we seem to be receiving a cloud of unprocessed information that is not in an order that we can easily assimilate.

These are very genuine concerns – there is no doubt that open methods do seem to produce a less ordered consultation. However, there is a way out of this important difficulty: *structuring the consultation via summary and signposting* provides an alternative method for the doctor to obtain order and appropriate control without sacrificing the benefits of openness. Summarizing as a structuring tool allows you to:

- pull together, review and remember what you have heard so far
- order the information into a coherent pattern
- realize what information you still need to obtain or clarify
- gain space to consider where the consultation should go next
- separate and consider both disease and illness.

Learners grappling with the techniques of open questions and attentive listening find summarizing especially useful – when unsure of what to ask next or what the patient has already said, summarize and play for time! The very act of summarizing and the patient's response will normally establish the most appropriate path forward without embarrassment or apparent loss of momentum.

Signposting

WHAT IS SIGNPOSTING?

Signposting is the twin skill of summarizing. After summarizing produces a 'yes' response from the patient, signposting is used to:

- make the progression from one section to another
- explain the rationale for the next section.

'You mentioned two areas there that are obviously important, the pain and how you are going to cope with John. Could I start by asking a few more questions about the pain that would help me understand what might be causing it and then we can come back to your difficulties with John?'
or
'Since we haven't met before it will help me to learn something about your past medical history. Can we do that now?'
or
'I can see that you are in some discomfort but I need to ask a few questions about the drugs that your doctor has prescribed and then make a brief examination to be able to help sort out what exactly is going on.'

Use signposting to move from one section to the next so that:

- the patient understands where the interview is going and why
- you can share your thoughts and needs with the patient
- you can ask permission
- the consultation is structured overtly for you both.

Examples of when to signpost during history taking include when moving:

- from the introduction into the information-gathering stage
- from open to closed questions
- into specific questions about the patient's ideas, concerns or expectations
- into different parts of the history (e.g. from present to past history)
- into the physical examination
- into explanation and planning.

Summarizing and signposting together provide an overt structure apparent to the patient; the patient understands and becomes part of the structuring process. This is so much better than structure via the use of closed questions where the patient is left in the dark about the process of the interview.

Another of the five principles of effective communication that we discussed in Chapter 1 is *reducing unnecessary uncertainty*. Unresolved uncertainties can lead to lack of concentration or anxiety which in turn can block effective communication. By knowing where the interview is going and why, much possible uncertainty and anxiety is reduced – in the case above, the patient knows that you have picked up her cue about her husband and that there will be an opportunity to explore this in a little while. This frees her to concentrate on the next part of the interview without worrying that one of her main concerns might not be addressed.

Levinson *et al.* (1997) showed that primary care physicians who used more signposting, which was described in this study as 'orientating statements', were less likely to have suffered malpractice claims.

Summarizing and signposting together therefore:

- are key skills promoting a collaborative and interactive interview
- make the structure overt and understood to the patient
- allow you and the patient to know where you are going and why
- allow you to signal a change in direction
- establish mutually understood common ground and reduce uncertainty for the patient.

SWANSEA PSYCHIATRIC EDUCATION LIBRARY

Sequencing

After agenda setting and negotiation have established an overt and mutually agreed plan for the interview, it is clearly the responsibility of the clinician to help carry out the plan and maintain a logical *sequence* which is apparent to the patient as the interview unfolds. A flexible but ordered approach to organization, with clear transitions from one section of the interview to the next, helps both physician and patient in efficient and accurate data gathering.

Cassata (1978), in his comments on structuring the interview, has emphasized the importance of two-way communication in each part of the consultation and, in particular, stresses the importance of making expectations and agendas overt. This encourages patient participation, ownership and collaboration. This process is enhanced and further encouraged by summarizing and signposting. So instead of ordering implicitly via closed questions, we recommend a pattern of structuring the consultation overtly via the following skills:

1 problem identification
2 screening
3 agenda setting
4 negotiation
5 internal summarizing
6 signposting
7 sequencing.

Summary

In this chapter, we have looked at both the theory and practice of gathering information. We have seen the strengths and limitations of the traditional method of history taking and the need for a transformed clinical method that takes into account both the doctor's and the patient's perspectives of the problem being discussed. We have seen that accurate and efficient information gathering is not achieved simply by interrogating the patient for symptoms but requires the more effective initial technique of open questions and listening. We have also seen the value of structuring the consultation in an overt fashion that encourages a collaborative interactional approach.

Before moving on to the physical examination or to the explanation and planning phase of the interview, the doctor needs to think through the skills outlined in the 'Gathering information' section of the *Calgary–Cambridge observation guide* and to consider: 'Have I explored the disease aspect of the patient's problems effectively; have I explored the patient's perspective of their problems and understood the meaning of the illness to the patient; have I ensured that the information gathered is accurate and complete; have I confirmed that I have understood the story correctly; have I continued to develop a supportive and collaborative environment?'. If so, she can move on with confidence.

4

Building the relationship

Introduction

We now consider the skills involved in building the relationship with the patient. In contrast to the other four sections of the interview which follow a natural sequence as the consultation evolves, building the relationship occurs throughout the interview. Building the relationship runs in parallel to the other tasks of the interview; it is the cement that binds the consultation together.

Beginning the consultation

Gathering information

⎫
⎬ Building the relationship
⎭

Explanation and planning

Closing the interview

Building the relationship is a task that is easily taken for granted or forgotten. The other components of the interview often dominate as doctors move through the consultation trying to make sense of the patient's illness and disease. Yet without paying specific attention to the skills of relationship building, these more 'concrete' tasks become much more difficult to achieve. Relationship building in the consultation can be an end in itself – the doctor's role is sometimes that of supportive counselling alone. But in the majority of consultations, relationship building is an essential means of achieving all three goals of medical communication: accuracy, efficiency and supportiveness. As we see in this chapter, relationship building enables the patient to tell their story and explain their own concerns, it promotes adherence and helps prevent misunderstanding and conflict.

Forging a relationship with the patient is central to the success of every consultation whatever the context. Often, especially in specialist medicine, the relationship between doctor and patient is short-term in nature. Here, developing rapport is of vital importance; it enables the patient to feel comfortable in discussing problems with an unfamiliar person and to benefit fully from the consultation. Yet the doctor faces the added difficulty of having to accomplish the task of relationship building in a short period of time and often in the face of considerable patient anxiety.

Building the relationship is also the entry point to a longer term view of medical practice than we have considered so far. In many circumstances, the relationship between doctor and patient extends beyond a single interview into a continuing association over many meetings (Leopold *et al.* 1996). The development of a trusting relationship over several years is seen by many doctors as the most rewarding aspect of their work.

Patients wish their doctors to be competent and knowledgeable but they also need to be able to relate to their doctor, to feel understood and to be supported through adversity. Attention to relationship building offers the potential prize of patients who are more satisfied with their doctors and doctors who feel less frustrated and more satisfied in their work (Levinson *et al.* 1993).

Problems in communication

There are considerable reports in the media of patient dissatisfaction with the doctor–patient relationship. Many articles comment on doctors' lack of understanding of the patient as a person with individual concerns and wishes. Perhaps most striking are those articles written by physicians themselves who have found themselves in the unexpected role of patient. Many such articles are now published in series such as 'Personal View' in the *British Medical Journal*. So often they focus on the sudden revelation of the inhumanity of medicine or the lack of caring and support offered by their physicians. What a shame that it takes our personal experience of illness to draw this to our attention.

From the very earliest research into medical communication, relationship problems have featured highly as predictors of poor outcome. In Korsch *et al.*'s (1968) seminal study of 800 visits to a paediatric walk-in out-patients in Los Angeles, physician lack of warmth and friendliness was one of the most important variables related to poor levels of patient satisfaction and compliance.

Poole and Sanson-Fisher (1979) have shown that there are significant problems in medical education in the development of relationship-building skills. They demonstrated that we cannot assume that doctors have the ability to communicate empathically with patients or that they will acquire this ability during their medical training. They demonstrated poor skills in empathy in both first and final year medical students. They also showed that psychiatric residents, who might be thought to develop these skills in their training, also demonstrated low empathy skills.

Many commentators link the poor development of doctors' relationship-building skills with the way that students and residents are taught to remain 'uninvolved' during their medical training. As we have seen in Chapter 3, the traditional clinical method based on scientific reasoning values clinical detachment. Medical students are brought up in the world of the objective and the technological. At the expense of understanding the sick person, they are taught to concentrate on underlying disease mechanisms. Much is made in traditional medical education of the need to protect ourselves from the powerful emotions of medical practice where feelings are painful for both patient and doctor. Impassive objectivity is recommended as a coping mechanism. In this milieu, relationship-building skills clearly will not flourish.

Objectives

The objectives that we seek to accomplish in building the relationship with the patient can be summarized as:

- developing rapport to enable the patient to feel understood, valued and supported
- encouraging an environment that maximizes accurate and efficient initiation, information gathering and explanation and planning
- enabling supportive counselling as an end in itself
- developing and maintaining a continuing relationship over time
- involving the patient so that he understands and is comfortable with the process of the consultation
- reducing potential conflict between doctor and patient
- increasing both the physician's and the patient's satisfaction with the consultation.

These objectives encompass many of the tasks and check-points mentioned in other well-known guides to the consultation:

Byrne and Long (1976)   Phase 1: the doctor establishes a relationship with the patient
Pendleton *et al.* (1984)   To establish or maintain a relationship with the patient
Neighbour (1987)   Connecting – establishing rapport with the patient
Cohen-Cole (1991)   Developing rapport and responding to the patient's emotions
Keller and Carroll (1994)   Engaging the patient
                               Empathizing with the patient.

'What' to teach and learn about building the relationship – the evidence for the skills

Next we examine in detail the individual skills for building the relationship, listed in Box 4.1, and explore the evidence from theory and research which validates their use in the consultation.

SECTION 1: NON-VERBAL COMMUNICATION

We cannot emphasize enough the importance of non-verbal communication throughout the medical interview. We need to pay as much attention to the effect of our non-verbal interaction

---

Box 4.1   Skills for building the relationship

Non-verbal communication

- **Demonstrates appropriate non-verbal behaviour:** e.g. eye contact, posture and position, movement, facial expression, use of voice
- **Use of notes:** if reads, writes notes or uses computer, does in a manner that does not interfere with dialogue or rapport
- **Picks up patient's non-verbal cues:** body language, speech, facial expression, affect; checks them out and acknowledges as appropriate

Developing rapport

- **Acceptance:** acknowledges patient's views and feelings; accepts legitimacy; is not judgemental
- **Empathy and support:** e.g. expresses concern, understanding, willingness to help; acknowledges coping efforts and appropriate self-care
- **Sensitivity:** deals sensitively with embarrassing and disturbing topics and physical pain, including when associated with physical examination

Involving the patient

- **Sharing of thoughts:** shares thinking with patient to encourage patient's involvement (e.g. 'What I'm thinking now is …')
- **Provides rationale:** explains rationale for questions or parts of physical examination that could appear to be non-sequiturs
- **Examination:** during physical examination, explains process, asks permission

---

with patients as we do to the impact of our words (Friedman 1979; Hall *et al.* 1995). Two intimately related aspects of non-verbal communication require consideration:

1 the non-verbal behaviour of patients
2 the non-verbal behaviour of doctors.

As doctors, we need to recognize patients' non-verbal cues in their speech patterns, facial expression, affect and body posture. But we also need to be aware of our own non-verbal behaviour, how the physician's use of eye contact, body position and posture, movement, facial expression and use of voice can all influence the success of the consultation. Box 4.2 clarifies what is meant by non-verbal communication.

What is the difference between verbal and non-verbal communications?

What are the differences between verbal and non-verbal communication (Verderber and Verderber 1980)?

Box 4.2   What do we mean by non-verbal communication?

- **Posture:** sitting, standing; erect, relaxed
- **Proximity:** use of space, physical distance between communicators
- **Touch:** handshake, pat, physical contact during physical examination
- **Body movements:** hand and arm gestures, fidgeting, nodding, foot and leg movements
- **Facial expression:** raised eyebrows, frown, smiles, crying
- **Eye behaviour:** eye contact, gaze, stares
- **Vocal cues:** pitch, rate, volume, rhythm, silence, pause, tone, speech errors, affect, responsiveness
- **Use of time:** early, late, on time, overtime, rushed, slow to respond
- **Physical presence:** race, gender, body shape, clothing, grooming
- **Environmental cues:** location, furniture placement, lighting, temperature, colour

---

- Verbal communication is discrete with clear endpoints – we know when the message has come to an end. In contrast, non-verbal communication is continuous – it goes on for as long as the communicators are in each other's presence. We cannot stop communicating non-verbally (Watzlawick *et al.* 1967); even when people are together in silence, the atmosphere is filled with messages. The difference between comfortable and uncomfortable silence is often mediated by our non-verbal communication.
- Verbal communication occurs in a single mode, either auditory (spoken) or visual (written), whereas non-verbal communication can occur in several modes at once. We can send and receive all the non-verbal cues listed in Box 4.2 simultaneously; all of our senses can be receiving signals at once.
- Verbal communication is mostly under voluntary control whereas non-verbal communication operates at the edge of or beyond our conscious awareness. Non-verbal communication can be amenable to deliberate control; for instance, we use non-verbal cues from voice, body, head and eye movement deliberately to help coordinate the taking of turns in conversation. However, non-verbal communication also operates at a less conscious level. Our non-verbal communication may be 'leaking' spontaneous clues to the receiver that we are not even aware of and may be providing a better representation of our true feelings than our more considered verbal comments. DiMatteo *et al.* (1980) have shown that this is particularly true for body posture and movement.
- Verbal messages are more effective in communicating discrete pieces of information and in conveying our intellectual ideas and thoughts. In contrast, non-verbal communication is the channel most responsible for communicating our attitudes, emotions and affect, for conveying the way we present ourselves and how we relate. Considerably more cues about liking, responsiveness and dominance are provided by non-verbal than verbal means. Non-verbal communication plays an increasingly important role when someone is unable or unwilling to explicitly express feelings verbally, for example when cultural taboos dictate against disagreeing with a superior or where words are inadequate to describe love or grief or pain (Ekman *et al.* 1972; Mehrabian 1972; Argyle 1975).

Why understanding non-verbal communication can make a difference in the consultation

Non-verbal communication can work to accent, qualify, regulate, take the place of or contradict verbal communication. In most circumstances, verbal and non-verbal communication work together to reinforce one another. Non-verbal cues enable verbal messages to be delivered more accurately and efficiently by strengthening the verbal message. For example, after the doctor has summarized and asked *'Have I got that right?'*, the patient says *'Yes, that's spot on'* and smiles, leans forward and uses an animated voice, or as the patient talks of her fears about her surgery, she looks down, talks more slowly and plays with her fingers.

When we are deprived of accompanying non-verbal confirmation, our verbal conversation is more liable to be misunderstood; we have all encountered problems communicating over the telephone where we are denied so many non-verbal cues.

We can intentionally use non-verbal communication to reduce uncertainty and misunderstanding in our verbal communication. *'Are you happy with that plan?'* accompanied by eye contact, hands opened out and an enquiring facial expression will indicate your genuine interest. Alternatively, the same phrase accompanied by a closure of the notes, hands banged on the table and a quick look at the patient and then away all suggests that you do not want to know if the answer is no.

As we can see from the last example, the two channels can also work to contradict each other. Communication research has shown that when the two are inconsistent or contradictory, non-verbal messages will override verbal messages (Koch 1971; McCroskey *et al.* 1971). If the verbal statement is *'Tell me about your problem'* while the non-verbal cues are speaking quickly and looking agitated, the patient will make the correct interpretation that time is at a premium today. If the doctor says there is nothing to worry about but hesitates in her speech as she delivers this verbal message, the patient will assume that perhaps there is some concern and that information is being withheld. However, this generalization may apply only to normal adults. Young children and emotionally disturbed adults or adolescents tend to believe the verbal message when faced with contradictions or inconsistencies (Reilly and Muzarkara 1978).

A further use of non-verbal behaviour relates to the reinforcement theory of social interaction (Mehrabian and Ksionsky 1974) and to non-verbal synchrony (DeVito 1988). People tend to act in ways which reinforce their general expectations. People also tend to mirror or imitate each other's non-verbal behaviour – to move or talk in synchronization – as a gesture of affiliation. Doctors can use these concepts to advantage first by anticipating a positive experience with their patients and second by modelling relaxed attentive listening skills. Unconscious mirroring and reinforcement of this behaviour by patients will enable them also to relax and become more attentive. We can affect others positively through our behaviour. On the other hand, if we are disinterested, our non-verbal behaviour will be picked up by the patient and communication can deteriorate.

What is the research evidence that non-verbal communication makes a difference to the consultation?

Harrigan *et al.* (1985) demonstrated that doctors who face their patients directly, have more eye contact and maintain open arm postures are regarded as more empathic, interested and warm.

Weinberger *et al.* (1981), in a study of hospital-based internal medicine out-patients, reported a positive relationship between patient satisfaction and physician non-verbal communication in the form of physician nods and gestures and closer distance between doctor and patient in the information-gathering phase.

Larsen and Smith (1981) demonstrated in family medicine that non-verbal immediacy, defined in terms of touch, closer distance, leaning forward, body orientation and gaze, is related to patient satisfaction as well as patient understanding.

Hall *et al.* (1981) used the technique of filtered speech to separate verbal messages from vocal cues: in electronically manipulated recordings, vocal expression could be heard but not the content of words. They showed in a family and community health clinic that patients and doctors reciprocated their emotions in their voice quality. If one party appeared satisfied or angry or anxious, so did the other. This reciprocation was far more apparent in filtered speech than in non-filtered speech or written transcripts. The authors inferred that much of the affective communication actively responded to in the interaction takes place via non-verbal cues. They also demonstrated a difference between verbal and non-verbal channels in relation to patient satisfaction. Verbal messages using words that appeared less anxious and more sympathetic were related to greater patient satisfaction. In contrast, non-verbal messages that were more angry or anxious also led to more patient satisfaction. Similar findings were demonstrated in relation to patient compliance in appointment keeping. The authors suggest that non-verbal cues of anger and anxiety are interpreted by the patient as reflecting concern and seriousness on the part of the physician. Clearly, the verbal and non-verbal channels offer very different information about affect.

Hall *et al.* (1987) demonstrated that doctors in primary care who were high information givers were also rated highly on their voice tone by independent observers; they were more interested, more anxious and less bored. In contrast, physicians who gave less information spent more time in pleasantries but had voices that were perceived as bored or calm. Again, the authors conclude that anxiety in the doctor's voice is perceived as anxious regard. This interpretation would fit well with the work of Kaplan *et al.* (1989) which we discuss in detail in Chapter 5. They found that 'negative affect' expressed by both physician and patient was related to better health outcomes. The authors concluded that this may represent 'healthy friction' or it may be that doctors who are more engaged with their patients appear more anxious or concerned.

DiMatteo *et al.* (1980; 1986) showed that internal medicine residents and family practice residents who rated highly on objective laboratory tests of their ability to communicate emotion through their faces and voices ('encoding') had patients who were more satisfied with their medical care and, interestingly, more patients on their lists! Physicians who tested highly on their ability to recognize the meanings of patients' non-verbal cues ('decoding') had more satisfied patients with better appointment keeping!

Goldberg *et al.* (1983) demonstrated that family practice residents who established eye contact were more likely to detect emotional distress in their patients.

What then are the lessons for physicians?

Physicians therefore need to be aware of both their patients' and their own non-verbal behaviour.

READING THE NON-VERBAL CUES OF PATIENTS

Being able to 'decode' non-verbal cues is essential if doctors wish to understand patients' feelings. The cultural norms of the health care setting militate against patients' expressing their feelings verbally – patients are often reluctant to express their thoughts or feelings openly but instead use covert messages (see p.109, Chapter 5). Non-verbal cues may therefore be one of the few indicators to the physician of a patient's desire to contribute their own concerns about a problem.

Just because spontaneous cues representing true feelings are being sent does not mean that you can interpret those cues accurately simply by noticing them – there are many sources of possible distortion and misunderstanding inherent in receiving non-verbal messages. To ensure accurate interpretation of such non-verbal behaviour, it is important not only to observe carefully but also to verify perceptions verbally. Your interpretations and assumptions may or may not be right; they need to be checked out with the patient. Checking your assumptions encourages patients to talk further about what they are thinking or feeling: it therefore has the double pay-off of both preventing possible misrepresentation and discovering more information.

The skills of picking up these cues and checking them out verbally (*'You seem upset – would you like to talk about it?'*) are described in Chapter 3.

Picking up on non-verbal cues not only helps the doctor to understand the emotional impact of the patient's illness but is also of considerable diagnostic importance in its own right. Reading the non-verbal cues of depression is an essential part of diagnosing the illness itself (Hall *et al.* 1995), while emotional problems only hinted at through non-verbal channels are often the root cause of physical symptoms.

TRANSMITTING YOUR OWN NON-VERBAL CUES

Similarly, without attention to your own non-verbal communication skills and the messages that you are transmitting through the non-verbal channel ('encoding'), much of your other efforts to communicate may be undone. If your verbal and non-verbal signals are contradictory, at the very least you risk confusion or misinterpretation, at worst your non-verbal message will win out. Non-verbal skills signalled through eye contact, posture, position, movement, facial expression, timing and voice can assist in demonstrating attentiveness to the patient and facilitate the formation of a helping relationship; ineffective attending behaviour, in contrast, closes off the interaction and prohibits relationship building (Gazda *et al.* 1995). Again, the disparity in power and control between patient and doctor leads patients to be particularly attentive to non-verbal cues to doctors' attitudes and meanings; patients rarely ask for verbal confirmation of cues that they pick up and commonly base their impressions on non-verbal messages alone.

Use of notes and records

One of the most important of all non-verbal skills is eye contact. Yet so often, doctors refer to the patient's written or computer record during the consultation while the patient is speaking and lose eye contact. Heath (1984), in a qualitative study in British general practice, examined the consequences of physicians attempting to read the patient's records and listen to the patient at the same time. She demonstrated how instead of increasing efficiency, quite the opposite occurs:

- patients withhold their initial reply to the doctor's solicitation until eye contact is given
- patients pause in mid-utterance when the doctor looks at the notes and resume when eye contact is regained
- patients use body movement to catch the doctor's gaze if he is reading the notes while the patient is talking
- patients' fluency deteriorates as the doctor looks away and recovers on re-establishment of gaze
- doctors frequently miss or forget information given to them while they are reading their notes.

Eye contact allows the patient to infer that the doctor is prepared to participate and listen. Without established eye contact, the patient makes non-verbal efforts to encourage the doctor to realign his gaze and there is a reduction in quality and quantity of information provided.

The conclusion of this study is that using records while the patient is speaking is not an efficient way of conducting the consultation for either patient or doctor. The patient will give their information more slowly and less completely and the doctor may well not 'hear' the information provided. Heath suggests various strategies to overcome the common problem of needing to both hear the patient's story and examine their records:

- deliberately postpone using the records until the patient has completed their opening statement
- wait for opportune moments before looking at the notes
- separate listening from note reading by verbally signposting both your intention to look at the records and when you have finished, so that the patient understands the process.

SECTION 2: DEVELOPING RAPPORT

Acceptance

In Chapter 3, we looked at the importance of understanding the patient's perspective. We examined the need to elicit patients' *thoughts* (their ideas, concerns and expectations) and take note of their *feelings*. But having discovered these thoughts and feelings, how should doctors respond? The concept of acceptance, as proposed by Briggs and Banahan (1979), is helpful here. It suggests that instead of immediate reassurance, rebuttal or even agreement, one of the most useful initial responses to patients' contributions is to give an 'accepting response'.

THE ACCEPTING RESPONSE

Also called the 'supportive response' or the 'acknowledging response' elsewhere in the literature, the accepting response provides a practical and specific way of:

- accepting non-judgementally what the patient says
- acknowledging the legitimacy of the patient to hold their own views and feelings
- valuing the patient's contributions.

The accepting response acknowledges and accepts both the patient and the patient's emotions or thoughts, wherever and whatever they are. This approach is effective in relationship building because it establishes common ground between doctor and patient through a shared understanding of the patient's perspective. Acceptance is at the root of trust and trust is the bedrock of successful relationships (Gibb 1961; Briggs and Banahan 1979).

Accepting patients' ideas and emotions without initial judgement may not be easy – especially if they do not accord with your own perceptions. But by acknowledging and valuing the patient's point of view rather than countering immediately with your own ideas, you can support the patient and enhance your relationship. The key concept here is acknowledging patients' rights to hold their own views and feelings. It helps for patients to understand that it is not only reasonable for them to have thoughts and emotions about their illnesses but it is also important to you as a doctor for these to be expressed so that you can appreciate their perspective and be aware of their needs.

FUNCTIONS OF THE ACCEPTING RESPONSE

The accepting response has three valuable functions:

1 to respond supportively to the patient's expression of feelings or thoughts
2 to act as a facilitative response to obtain a better understanding of these thoughts and feelings
3 to value the patient and their ideas even when their feelings or concerns seem unjustified or perhaps even wrong.

SKILLS OF THE ACCEPTING RESPONSE

The following set of skills can be used in the sequence shown below to signal acceptance to the patient. In this example, the patient has expressed his thoughts by saying *'I think I might have cancer, doctor; I've been getting an awful lot of wind lately'*:

• acknowledge the patient's thought or feeling by naming, restating or summarizing: *'So, you're worried that the wind might be caused by cancer.'*
• acknowledge the patient's right to feel or think as he does by using legitimizing comments: *'I can understand that you would want to get that checked out.'*
• come to a 'full stop'; use attentive silence and appropriate non-verbal behaviour to enable the patient to say more: *'Yes, doctor. You see, my mother died of bowel cancer when she was 40 and I remember she had a lot of wind – I'm terrified of getting it too.'*
• avoid the tendency to counter with *'yes, but …'*.

Although not a necessary part of every accepting response, it can also be helpful to:

• acknowledge the value to the doctor of the patient expressing their views: *'Thank you for telling me that. It's very helpful to know your concerns.'*

Responding to overt feelings and emotions
In the example above, we use the accepting response to respond to a patient's belief. Acceptance is equally valuable as an initial response to feelings and emotions. For instance, consider this accepting response to a bereaved patient saying of her dead husband *'I'm so angry with him. How could he have left me alone like that; he didn't even make a will'*.

'So, you feel angry about being left alone and about the will. I can see that must be upsetting.'
(Pause)
'Yes, I am. I'm so alone and I get so cross with him for not being with me and then I feel guilty for being angry with him. Am I going mad, doctor?'
'Those are strong emotions to deal with. I'm glad you mentioned them.'

Responding to indirectly expressed feelings and emotions
The next two examples demonstrate that the accepting response can be useful when the feeling or thought is indirectly expressed, for instance through non-verbal behaviour alone. Here we can combine picking up a cue to the patient's feelings (as we discussed in Chapter 3) with the accepting response:

'I sense that you feel uneasy about having to come to see me [the doctor is a haematologist] ... That's OK, many people feel that way when they first come here.' (Pause)
or
'I can see you're delighted with these test results; I'm glad they're so good too.' (Pause)

An important part of the accepting response is to come to a full stop after giving the initial acknowledgement, to wait briefly and attentively in silence and to avoid saying 'yes, but ...' which automatically negates the acceptance. This is almost a knee-jerk reaction for most of us. We are so eager to help that instead of waiting we say 'yes, but ...' and go on to give our point of view or correction to erroneous thinking or our reassurance before we give the patient a chance to feel the acceptance or to say anything further. All of this can come later, perhaps considerably later in the interview, *after* the patient has had an opportunity to respond to our statement of acceptance. It is of course imperative that we correct, advise and reassure; the question is when. What happens if we pause before we add the 'but ...' clause? Usually patients will respond with a brief outpouring of whatever thought or feeling has been acknowledged, share the burden or exhilaration and get it 'back' to a less overwhelming perspective so that they can talk about it further or go on to focus on other matters.

ACCEPTANCE IS NOT AGREEMENT

It is important to differentiate acceptance from agreement. Acknowledging that a patient would like further surgery is not the same as agreeing to perform it. It is a two-stage process. First, identify and acknowledge a patient's beliefs without immediately countering; this enables you to understand the patient without provoking initial defensiveness. If the patient's thoughts do not fit with your own, later on in the consultation and after due consideration go to the second stage: offer your own perspective and correct misapprehensions. Consider, for instance, if the patient in the example given above were a 20-year-old man. Contrast the following possible replies to his statement 'I think I might have cancer, doctor; I've been getting an awful lot of wind lately':

'Oh, we all get wind but that's not a sign of cancer at your age, what exactly have you noticed?'
'Well, I've just felt more blown up after meals and keep passing wind in the evenings.'
'That doesn't sound like anything to worry about.'

This approach devalues the importance of the patient's views and although most probably correct, the reassurance comes too early in the consultation to be accepted by the patient. The patient will not be encouraged to propose his own theories in the future. Instead, we could follow the plan proposed earlier:

'So, you're worried that the wind might be caused by cancer.' (Pause)
'Yes doctor. You see, my mother died of bowel cancer when she was 40 and I remember she had a lot of wind.'
'I can understand your concern – we'll check that out carefully. Tell me a bit more about your symptoms and then I'll examine you to see if you're OK.'

Here, instead of countering the patient's view or giving premature reassurance, the importance to you of hearing the patient's concerns is emphasized. You can explain and correct misconceptions later.

Acceptance is the second stage in the three-stage process of discovering patients' beliefs that we introduced in Chapter 3:

1 **identification** – discover and listen to the patient's ideas, concerns and expectations
2 **acceptance** – acknowledge the patient's views and their right to hold them, without necessarily agreeing with them
3 **explanation** – explain your understanding of the problem in relation to the patient's understanding and reach mutually understood common ground.

Acceptance makes it possible for doctors to remain open to their patients. It precludes judgemental remarks. It reinforces a tentative frame of mind, prevents premature closure or defensive reactions and instead establishes mutual common ground. It is this that ultimately allows for change.

THE PROBLEM OF PREMATURE REASSURANCE

Acceptance also gives us a way to avoid the trap of premature reassurance. Simple reassurance by itself may not be an effective supportive response (Wasserman *et al.* 1984). Often reassurance is given before adequate information has been obtained, before the patient's concerns have been discovered and before rapport has been developed. Unless we obtain sufficient information first, reassurance may sound false. Unless we understand the patient's fears, we may be addressing the wrong concern. Unless we have developed rapport with the patient, reassurance may well be interpreted as indifference or as being dismissive. And lastly, unless appropriate and relevant information is provided to back up our reassurance, the patient will not understand the basis for our assertions (Kessel 1979). Acceptance prevents premature reassurance – by discovering and accepting the patient's concerns, trust is developed and more information can be obtained about the patient's illness and their concerns before an opinion is offered. Reassurance when it comes can then be appropriately timed, properly explained and matched to the patient's concerns.

Before we have collected further information or ordered tests we may not be in a position to provide reassurance that there is nothing to worry about. But we still have much to offer. We can accept the patient's concern and then use reassurance in other more appropriate ways. Instead of reassuring about the disease, we can, for instance, reassure the patient about our intent: we can offer our support by demonstrating that we wish to work with the patient and that we will give careful attention to their concerns.

Empathy

One of the key skills in building the doctor–patient relationship is the use of empathy (Spiro 1992). Of all the skills in the consultation, this is the one most often thought by learners to be a matter of personality rather than skill. Although some of us may naturally be better at demonstrating empathy than others, the skills of empathy, like any other communication skill, can be learned. The challenge is to identify the building blocks of the empathic response and enable learners to integrate the elements of empathy into their natural style so that it appears genuine to both doctor and patient (Platt and Keller 1994; Gazda *et al*. 1995).

Empathy is a two-stage process:

1 the understanding and sensitive appreciation of another person's predicament or feelings
2 the communication of that understanding back to the patient in a supportive way.

The key to empathy is not only being sensitive but overtly demonstrating that sensitivity to the patient so that they appreciate your understanding and support. It is not good enough to think empathically, you must show it too. Empathy demonstrated in this way overcomes the isolation of the individual in their illness and is strongly therapeutic in its own right. It also acts as a strong facilitative opening, enabling the patient to divulge more of their thoughts and concerns. What, then, are the building blocks of the empathic response?

UNDERSTANDING THE PATIENT'S PREDICAMENT AND FEELINGS

Many of the skills that we discuss throughout this book demonstrate to patients that we are genuinely interested in hearing about their thoughts. Together these skills provide an atmosphere which facilitates disclosure and enables the first step of empathy, understanding the patient's predicament, to take place:

- welcoming the patient warmly
- clarifying the patient's agenda and expectations
- attentive listening
- facilitation, especially via paraphrasing of content and feelings and repetition
- encouraging the expression of feelings and thoughts
- picking up cues, checking out our interpretations or assumptions
- summarizing
- acceptance
- non-judgemental response
- use of silence
- encouraging the patient to contribute as an equal
- offering choices.

Having set up a climate conducive to patient disclosure, the doctor has to pick up patients' verbal and non-verbal cues, become aware of their predicament and consider their feelings and emotions.

COMMUNICATING EMPATHY TO THE PATIENT

The skills outlined above do not complete the second stage of empathy, communicating your understanding back to the patient so that they know you appreciate and are sensitive to their difficulty. Both non-verbal and verbal skills can help us here.

Empathic non-verbal communication can say more than a thousand words. Facial expression, proximity, touch, tone of voice or use of silence in response to a patient's expression of feelings can clearly signal to the patient that you are sensitive to their predicament. But what are the verbal skills that allow you to demonstrate empathy? Empathic statements are supportive comments that specifically link the 'I' of the doctor and the 'you' of the patient. They both name and appreciate the patient's affect or predicament (Platt and Keller 1994):

- 'I can see that your husband's memory loss has been very difficult for **you** to cope with.'
- 'I can appreciate how difficult it is for **you** to talk about this.'
- 'I can sense how angry **you** have been feeling about your illness.'
- 'I can see that **you** have been very upset by her behaviour.'
- 'I can understand that it must be frightening for **you** to know the pain might keep coming back.'

It is not necessary to have shared an experience to empathize, nor to feel yourself that you would find that experience hard. It is necessary, however, to see the problem *from the patient's position* and communicate your understanding back to the patient. Empathy should not be confused with sympathy which is a feeling of pity or concern from *outside the patient's position*.

Poole and Sanson-Fisher (1979) have clearly shown that empathy is a construct that can be learned. They utilized a nine-point evaluation scale, developed by Truax and Carkhuff (1967), which ranges from stage 1: 'completely unaware of even the most conspicuous of the client's statements; responses not appropriate to the mood and content of the client's statements' to stage 9: 'unerringly responds to the client's full range of feelings in their exact intensity; recognizes each emotional nuance and reflects them in his words and voice; expands the client's hints into a full-blown but tentative elaboration of feeling or experience with unerring sensitive accuracy'! Truax has shown that psychotherapists who score highly on this scale achieve change.

Poole and Sanson-Fisher showed that medical students' ability to empathize did not improve over their medical school career without specific training: both first and final year students scored poorly on the evaluation scale (average 2.1). However, after participating in eight two-hour workshops using audio-tapes, students' scale ratings significantly improved to an average level of 4.5 (stage 5: 'accurately responds to all the client's discernible feelings; any misunderstandings are not disruptive due to their tentative nature'). After training, students also:

- used less jargon
- made clear attempts to understand the unique meaning of events, words and symptoms to patients
- less often blocked off emotion-laden areas
- obtained descriptions of more of their patients' problem areas
- more often matched their voice tone to their patients'

- did less talking
- responded more in an understanding mode
- offered less advice
- were reported by patients to be understanding and caring.

Support

Several other supportive approaches contribute to rapport and relationship building (Rogers 1980; Egan 1990). They are often used to complete the empathic response:

- **concern:** 'I'm concerned that you'll be going home on your own tonight and might not be able to cope with your arm in a cast.'
- **understanding:** 'I can certainly understand how you might feel angry with the hospital for cancelling your operation.'
- **willingness to help:** 'If there is anything else I can do for Jack, please let me know' or 'Although as I say we can't cure the cancer, I can help with any symptoms that it might cause so please tell me straight away if anything happens.'
- **partnership:** 'We'll have to work together to get on top of this illness so let's work through the options that we can choose from.'
- **acknowledging coping efforts and appropriate self-care:** 'You've really done exactly the right things in trying to get his temperature down' or 'I think you've coped really well at home despite some very considerable problems.'
- **sensitivity:** 'I'm sorry if this examination is embarrassing for you. I'll try to make it as quick and easy as I can.'

The key point here is that your thoughts need to be verbalized to be supportive. Communication must be overt to be truly effective and not liable to misinterpretation. Without explicit comment, the patient may well not be fully aware of your support.

What is the research evidence that rapport-building skills make a difference to the medical consultation?

Buller and Buller (1987) described two general styles displayed by physicians in medical interviews. The first, affiliation, was composed of behaviours designed to establish and maintain a positive doctor–patient relationship. Many of these behaviours were those discussed in the section above, including friendliness, interest, attentiveness, empathy, non-judgemental attitude and social orientation. The second style included behaviours that established the doctor's power, status, authority and professional distance. Patient satisfaction was found to be significantly higher when doctors in both specialist and family practice adopted the affiliative style.

Bertakis *et al.* (1991), in a study of physicians from both internal medicine and family practice, demonstrated that patients are most satisfied by interviews that encourage them to talk about psychosocial issues in an atmosphere characterized by an absence of physician dominance and the presence of friendliness and interest.

Hall *et al.* (1988), in a meta-analysis of 41 independent studies, reported that patient satisfaction was related to the amount of information given by doctors, technical and interpersonal competence, more partnership building, more positive talk, more positive non-verbal behaviour and more social conversation. The definitions used to group behaviours together under 'partnership building' and 'positive talk' include many of the rapport-building skills discussed above.

Wasserman *et al.* (1984) analysed the effect of supportive statements made to mothers during paediatric visits. They found that empathic statements led to increased satisfaction and reduction in maternal concerns. Encouragement (such as acknowledging coping efforts and appropriate self-care) led to increased satisfaction and higher opinions of clinicians. In contrast, simple reassurance, which was the commonest intervention, led to no improvements in outcome. This confirms the suggestion that reassurance without understanding the patient's concerns or providing adequate information may be of little value.

Wissow *et al.* (1994) found that paediatricians' use of supportive statements (compliments, approval, concern, empathy, encouragement and reassurance) was positively associated with parents' disclosure of psychosocial problems.

Spiegel *et al.* (1989) conducted a longitudinal study of women with metastatic carcinoma of the breast, comparing a control group with a second group of women assigned to a year of weekly supportive-expressive group therapy. Women in the experimental group were encouraged to provide mutual support, express and discuss their feelings and concerns about dying, develop a life project for their remaining time, examine their relationships with others, work through doctor–patient problems and use self-hypnosis to aid pain control. After four years, all of the control-group patients had died and one-third of the experimental group were still alive. Over 10 years, women attending the support group had lived on average 18 months longer than women in the control group. Although this study looked at the effects of supportive group therapy rather than the doctor–patient relationship *per se*, we report this study here because it speaks to the importance of expressing feelings in a supportive climate and the power of relationship in health care. It also serves as a reminder that in addition to developing the best relationship possible with their patients, doctors can also point them in the direction of support groups and other professionals who can fulfil additional relationship needs.

SECTION 3: INVOLVING THE PATIENT

One of the principles of effective communication that we presented in Chapter 1 was *reducing unnecessary uncertainty*. Unresolved uncertainties can lead to lack of concentration or anxiety which in turn can block effective communication. For example, patients may be uncertain about what to expect during a given interview, about the significance of a line of questioning, about the role of a particular member of the health care team or about the attitudes, intentions or trustworthiness of the doctor. Therefore one important aspect of building the relationship in the consultation is to employ skills that limit the uncertainty that can so easily block communication.

Sharing of thoughts

Throughout this book, we espouse a system of medical communication that encourages a collaborative understanding between patient and doctor. We have seen how important it is for patient and doctor to understand each other and the steps that we can take to ensure that communication in the consultation is an interaction rather than a one-way transmission. Techniques such as *the use of summary* in information gathering and *checking understanding* in information giving not only ensure accuracy but also act as facilitative openings by encouraging a truly interactive process.

Sharing your thinking with the patient is another example of encouraging the patient's involvement:

'What I'm thinking now is how to sort out whether this arm pain is coming from your shoulder or your neck.'
or
'Sometimes it's difficult to work out whether abdominal pain is due to a physical illness or is related to stress.'

Sharing your thought processes in this way not only allows the patient to understand the reasons for your questions but also acts as a facilitative probe:

'I think you might be right about stress, doctor. I've had a terrible time with my son just recently and I just don't know how to cope.'

This overt approach allows the patient an insight into the process of the interview, enabling him to understand the drift of your questioning and providing a very open-ended method of eliciting further information. It is often more acceptable than thinking through the dilemma internally and then posing closed questions without explanation:

'Are you under any stress at the moment?'

Closed questions so often feel unsettling to the patient because of uncertainty about what lies behind the doctor's choice of direction:

'Does the doctor think I'm just neurotic?'

Providing a rationale

Explaining the rationale for questions or parts of the physical examination is another specific example of the principle of reducing uncertainty. Many questions and examinations remain a mystery to the patient unless explained. For example, when taking a history from a patient with chest pain, doctors commonly ask:

'How many pillows do you sleep with?'

This appears to the patient to be a complete non-sequitur. Why is the doctor asking him about his bedtime habits? Yet the doctor could so easily have asked:

'Do you get breathless when you lie flat at night?'
followed if necessary by
'Do you have to prop yourself up on several pillows?'

Similarly, without explaining why they are performing parts of the examination, doctors can leave the patient in confusion and may even lay themselves open to medico-legal attack. The young female patient who comes in with a sore throat will be surprised if the male doctor starts to examine her groins unless he explains that she might have glandular fever and that he wishes to check for enlarged lymph glands. The man with sciatica may be worried by the doctor who starts to test perineal sensation with a pin unless the doctor explains about the danger of central prolapsed discs. Both these examples have led to formal complaints against doctors. Reducing uncertainty can decrease anxiety for the doctor too!

During physical examination, asking permission to perform each task is not only a matter of common courtesy but demonstrates to the patient that you are sensitive to their potential discomfiture and therefore promotes relationship building.

Summary

In this chapter, we have examined the skills of building the relationship, a task that is central to the success of the consultation. Without attention to both our own and our patients' non-verbal communication, without efforts to develop rapport and without taking pains to involve the patient in the process of the consultation, many problems will arise. Not only will our long-term relationship with the patient suffer, but even in the short term our patients will feel less understood and supported, the other tasks of the interview will become much more difficult to achieve and patient satisfaction and adherence will diminish.

Throughout the interview, the doctor has to pay specific attention to the skills of relationship building while completing the more sequential tasks of the consultation. By keeping in mind the skills outlined in this section of the *Calgary–Cambridge observation guide*, the doctor will be rewarded with a more accurate, efficient and supportive consultation that paves the way for the development of a trusting and productive long-term relationship.

5

Explanation and planning

Introduction

Explanation and planning is the Cinderella subject of communication skills teaching. Most teaching programmes concentrate on the first half of the interview and tend to neglect or underplay this vital next stage in the consultation (Maguire *et al.* 1986; Sanson-Fisher *et al.* 1991). To some extent, this emphasis is understandable as so many problems in communication arise from the beginning or information-gathering phases of the interview. Also, as we show in this chapter, many of the skills of successful explanation and planning are inextricably linked with the skills of information gathering – effective explanation needs both to be based on information gathered about the disease aspects of a patient's problems and also to be framed in terms that take into account the patient's illness framework of ideas, concerns and expectations.

Yet explanation and planning are of utmost importance to a successful consultation. There is little point in being able to discover what the patient wishes to discuss, in taking a good history and in being highly knowledgeable if you cannot make a joint management plan that the patient understands, feels comfortable with and is prepared to adhere to. Prescribing treatment that is not taken wastes all our efforts in assessment and diagnosis.

If the first half of the consultation represents the foundations of medical communication, explanation and planning are the roof. Neglecting this aspect may ruin all the hard work already expended on understanding the patient's problems.

Problems in communication

Research identifies substantial difficulties in the explanation and planning phase of the interview. In fact, the statistics concerning these problems pose worrying questions about the value of much of our everyday activities! Here we provide just a few examples from a large body of evidence.

Are there problems with the amount of information that doctors give?

Many studies show that in general physicians give sparse information to their patients:

- Waitzkin (1984) demonstrated that American internists devoted little more than one minute on average to the task of information giving in interviews lasting 20 minutes and over-estimated the amount of time that they spent on this task by a factor of nine
- Makoul *et al.* (1995) found that doctors in British general practice overestimated the extent to which they accomplished the following key tasks in explanation and planning: discussing the risks of medication, discussing the patient's ability to follow the treatment plan and eliciting the patient's opinion about medication prescribed
- Boreham and Gibson (1978), in a study in Australian general practice, showed that despite a lack of basic knowledge prior to the consultation and a strongly expressed desire to gain information concerning their illness, the majority of patients did not obtain even basic information concerning the diagnosis, prognosis, causation or treatment of their condition
- Svarstad (1974) studied doctors' instructions to patients when prescribing drugs and found no discussion at all in 20% of cases, no information about the name or purpose of the drug in 30%, no mention of the frequency of doses in 80% or the length of the course in 90%.

Are there problems with the type of information that doctors give?

We also know that patients and doctors disagree over the relative importance of different types of medical information:

- Kindelan and Kent (1987), in a study in British general practice, showed that patients placed the highest value on information about diagnosis, prognosis and causation of their condition. Doctors, however, greatly underestimated their patients' desire for information about prognosis and causation and overestimated their desire for information concerning treatment and drug therapy. Patients' individual information needs were not elicited.

Can patients understand the language that doctors use?

Many studies have shown that doctors not only use language that patients do not understand but also appear to use it to control their patients' involvement in the interview:

- Korsch *et al.* (1968) found that paediatricians' use of technical language (e.g. 'oedema') and medical shorthand (e.g. 'history') was a barrier to communication in more than half of the 800 visits studied. Mothers were confused by the terms used by doctors yet rarely asked for clarification of unfamiliar terms
- Svarstad (1974) suggested that doctors and patients engage in a 'communication conspiracy'. In only 15% of visits where unfamiliar terms were used did the patient admit that they did not understand. Doctors in turn seemed to speak as if their patients understood all that they said. Physicians deliberately used highly technical language to control communication and to limit patient questions – such behaviour occurred twice as often when doctors were under pressure of time
- McKinlay (1975), in a study of British obstetricians and gynaecologists, showed that physicians were well aware of the difficulties patients had in understanding doctors in general.

Despite this, in their interviews with patients, physicians continued to use terms which they had previously identified as the very ones that they would not expect their patients to understand.

DO PATIENTS RECALL AND UNDERSTAND THE INFORMATION THAT WE GIVE?

It is clear that patients do not recall all that we impart nor do they make sense of difficult messages. As we shall see later, early studies showed that only 50–60% of information given is recalled. Later studies have suggested that in fact much more is remembered and that the real difficulty is that patients do not always understand the meaning of key messages nor are they necessarily committed to the doctor's view.

DO PATIENTS COMPLY OR ADHERE TO THE PLANS THAT WE MAKE?

Here the research is clear-cut and salutary:

- studies have consistently shown that between 10% and 90% (with an average of 50%) of patients prescribed drugs by their doctors do not take their medicine at all or take it incorrectly
- many studies show that patients do not follow their doctors' recommendations, with 20–30% non-adherence in medications for acute illness, 30–40% in medications for illness prevention, 50% for long-term medications and 72% for diet
- yet surprisingly, doctors have a tendency to ignore non-compliance as a possible cause of poor outcome
- non-compliance is enormously expensive to the nation. Walton *et al.* in 1980 estimated that the cost of such wasted drugs per year in the UK was in the order of £300 million; more recent estimates of the overall costs of non-compliance (including extra visits to physicians, laboratory tests, additional medications, hospital and nursing home admissions, lost productivity and premature death) are CAN$7–9 billion in Canada (Coambs *et al.* 1995) and US$100 billion plus in the USA (Berg *et al.* 1993).

For further information about non-adherence, the following texts provide excellent reviews of the field: Haynes *et al.* (1979), Meichenbaum and Turk (1987), Ley (1988), Coambs *et al.* (1995) and Butler *et al.* (1996).

ARE THERE PROBLEMS 'N THE TEACHING OF EXPLANATION AND PLANNING IN MEDICAL EDUCATION?

Maguire *et al.* (1986) looked at the information-giving skills of young doctors who five years previously had completed training in interviewing skills at medical school. This training had, however, not included any specific training in information giving *per se*. The results were disturbing. Doctors were weakest in many of the very techniques which have been found to increase patients' satisfaction and compliance with advice and treatment:

- discovering the patient's views and expectations (70% no attempt)
- negotiation (90% no attempt)
- encouraging questions (70% no attempt)

- repetition of advice (63% no attempt)
- checking understanding (89% no attempt)
- categorizing information (90% no attempt).

No difference at all was detected in information-giving skills between those who had completed the course on interviewing skills at medical school and controls. Yet the same students had maintained their superiority over controls in key information-gathering skills (which have been the focus of their course). This demonstrates the need for teaching not only in information-gathering skills but also in the specific skills of explanation and planning if we wish doctors to become effective in information transfer in the consultation. Sanson-Fisher *et al.* (1991) have since argued that training medical practitioners in information transfer is the new challenge in communication skills teaching.

Objectives

Our objectives for this part of the interview can be summarized as:

- gauging the correct amount and type of information to give to each individual patient
- providing explanations that the patient can remember and understand
- providing explanations that relate to the patient's illness framework
- using an interactive approach to ensure a shared understanding of the problem with the patient
- involving the patient and planning collaboratively to increase the patient's commitment and adherence to plans made
- continuing to build a relationship and provide a supportive environment.

These objectives encompass many of the tasks and check-points mentioned in other well-known guides to the consultation:

Byrne and Long (1976)	Phase 4: the doctor, or the doctor and the patient, or the patient (in that order of probability) consider the condition
	Phase 5: the doctor and occasionally the patient detail further treatment or further investigation
Pendleton *et al.* (1984)	To choose with the patient an appropriate action for each problem
	To achieve a shared understanding of the problems with the patient
	To involve the patient in the management and encourage him to accept appropriate responsibility
	To establish and maintain a relationship with the patient
Neighbour (1987)	Handing over – doctor's and patient's agendas are agreed; negotiating, influencing and gift-wrapping
Cohen-Cole (1991)	Education, negotiation and motivation
	Developing rapport and responding to the patient's emotions
Keller and Carroll (1994)	Educating the patient
	Enlisting the patient in their own health care

'What' to teach and learn about explanation and planning – the evidence for the skills

Throughout Chapter 5, we examine in detail the individual skills for explanation and planning, listed in Box 5.1, and explore the evidence from theory and research which validates their use in the consultation.

Box 5.1   Skills for explanation and planning

Providing the correct amount and type of information

Aims: to give comprehensive and appropriate information; to assess each individual patient's information needs; to neither restrict or overload

- **Chunks and checks:** gives information in assimilable chunks; checks for understanding, uses patient's response as a guide to how to proceed
- **Assesses patient's starting point:** asks for patient's prior knowledge early on when giving information; discovers extent of patient's wish for information
- **Asks patients what other information would be helpful:** e.g. aetiology, prognosis
- **Gives explanation at appropriate times:** avoids giving advice, information or reassurance prematurely

Aiding accurate recall and understanding

Aims: to make information easier for the patient to remember and understand

- **Organizes explanation:** divides into discrete sections, develops a logical sequence
- **Uses explicit categorization or signposting:** e.g. 'There are three important things that I would like to discuss.'; 'Now, shall we move on to …'
- **Uses repetition and summarizing**: to reinforce information
- **Language:** uses concise, easily understood statements; avoids or explains jargon
- **Uses visual methods of conveying information:** diagrams, models, written information and instructions
- **Checks patient's understanding of information given (or plans made):** e.g. by asking patient to restate in own words; clarifies as necessary

Achieving a shared understanding: incorporating the patient's perspective

Aims: to provide explanations that relate to the patient's perspective of the problem; to discover the patient's thoughts and feelings about the information given; to encourage an interaction rather than one-way transmission

- **Relates explanations to patient's illness framework:** to previously elicited ideas, concerns and expectations
- **Provides opportunities and encourages patient to contribute:** to ask questions, seek clarification or express doubts; responds appropriately
- **Picks up verbal and non-verbal cues:** e.g. patient's need to contribute information or ask questions, information overload; distress
- **Elicits patient's beliefs, reactions and feelings:** re information given, terms used; acknowledges and addresses where necessary

Box 5.1 *Continued*

Planning: shared decision making

Aims: to allow patients to understand the decision-making process; to involve patients in decision making to the level they wish; to increase patients' commitment to plans made

- **Shares own thoughts:** ideas, thought processes and dilemmas
- **Involves patient by making suggestions** rather than directives
- **Encourages patient to contribute their thoughts:** ideas, suggestions and preferences
- **Negotiates a mutually acceptable plan**
- **Offers choices:** encourages patient to make choices and decisions to the level they wish
- **Checks with patient:** if accepts plans; if concerns have been addressed

Options in explanation and planning

If offering an opinion and discussing the significance of problems:

- **Offers opinion of what is going on and names if possible**
- **Reveals rationale for opinion**
- **Explains causation, seriousness, expected outcome, short- and long-term consequences**
- **Elicits patient's beliefs, reactions and concerns:** e.g. if opinion matches patient's thoughts; acceptability; feelings

If negotiating a mutual plan of action:

- **Discusses options:** e.g. no action, investigation, medication or surgery, non-drug treatments (physiotherapy, walking aids, fluids, counselling), preventative measures
- **Provides information on action or treatment offered:** name; steps involved, how it works; benefits and advantages; possible side-effects
- **Obtains patient's view of need for action, perceived benefits, barriers, motivation**
- **Accepts patient's views; advocates alternative viewpoint as necessary**
- **Elicits patient's reactions and concerns about plans and treatments:** acceptability
- **Takes patient's lifestyle, beliefs, cultural background and abilities into consideration**
- **Encourages patient to be involved in implementing plans, to take responsibility and be self-reliant**
- **Asks about patient support systems; discusses other support available**

If discussing investigations and procedures:

- **Provides clear information on procedures:** including what patient might experience and how patient will be informed of results
- **Relates procedures to treatment plan:** value and purpose
- **Encourages questions about and discussion of potential anxieties or negative outcomes**

SECTION 1: PROVIDING THE CORRECT AMOUNT AND TYPE
OF INFORMATION

One of the key issues of explanation and planning is how to gauge just what information to share with the patient. How do we negotiate the delicate path between not giving enough information and overloading the patient with too much?

Do patients and doctors agree over the amount of information that should be imparted?

We have already seen that there are problems with the amount of information doctors give to patients. But do patients wish to be better informed?

Doctors frequently misperceive the amount of information that their patients want, with a consistent tendency to underestimate the amount of information required. Waitzkin (1984) showed that in 65% of encounters, internists underestimated their particular patient's desire for information; in only 6% did they overestimate.

Faden *et al.* (1981) looked at the differences between attitudes of neurologists and their epileptic patients to the disclosure of information. They found that patients preferred to receive detailed disclosure of almost all risks associated with medication, even those that were quite rare. Physicians, however, said they were likely to disclose only those risks with a high probability of occurrence. Physicians felt that detailed disclosure of information about drugs would decrease compliance. Patients felt that disclosure would improve their compliance.

Many studies have shown that with the best of intentions, physicians choose to withhold information in an attempt to protect patients from worry. Pinder (1990) found that on making a diagnosis of Parkinson's disease, family doctors were most concerned with issues of 'protection': deciding how, when and whom to tell and deciding just how much to share about the diagnosis and prognosis. Patients, on the other hand, were attempting to comprehend and adjust to their illness, with many questions in their minds about the course of the disease and possible treatments, and many fears about the illness and their future prospects. Doctors tended to be positive, over-optimistic and protective. For instance, they avoided detail about drugs, were low-key about side-effects and did not explore the problems of long-term use of anti-Parkinsonian medication. Patients on average wanted to be given information and not be protected. Most patients wanted to understand their drugs and be forewarned about side-effects.

If the research shows that in general patients want more information (Cassileth *et al.* 1980; Beisecker and Beisecker 1990), why do doctors persist in giving them less? Why is there such a wide gulf between what doctors think patients want and what patients tell us they need? And how can doctors determine just how much information each individual patient would like? Much of the disparity between the amount of information that doctors give and the amount patients would prefer to receive has its roots in the traditional view of the doctor–patient relationship. In Chapter 3, we contrasted the traditional method of history taking with the disease–illness model of Western Ontario. We now take a similar approach to explanation and planning by comparing the traditional view of information giving with more modern concepts that mirror changes in society as a whole.

The traditional view of the doctor–patient relationship

AN UNBRIDGEABLE COMPETENCE GAP

The traditional view of the doctor–patient relationship held in the first part of this century was of an unbridgeable competence gap which made it impossible to achieve any semblance of true patient understanding. Parsons (1951) felt that doctors' vast training and knowledge created such a difference between them and their patients that it was not possible to explain complex issues appropriately. Patients simply acquiesced to their doctors' advice because of faith in their doctor as a person and in the medical profession as a whole. In this theory, patients relied on the wisdom of their doctor and were safeguarded by the profession's strong code of ethics which compelled the physician to act in the patient's best interests.

In this analysis, the medical consultation is somehow different from other situations where experts convey and share information with less expert clients – the specialist advising the general practitioner, the lawyer advising the house-purchaser, the scientist collaborating with the businessman, the teacher instructing students. In all of these situations, people with different levels of understanding and knowledge have to try to reach a compromise; sufficient information has to be imparted to allow successful communication and to enable clients to make informed choices and plans without being confused by excessive detail.

THE EMOTIONAL NATURE OF ILLNESS

So what is so different in the medical consultation to justify Parson's viewpoint? One argument used is that the highly emotional nature of illness prevents rational communication and understanding. It is suggested that the anxiety and fear of being placed in the patient role make patients passive, adopt a dependent 'sick' role and be willing to accept a well-intentioned, paternalistic medical adviser. By adopting the privileges of illness and convalescence, the patient is excused from everyday responsibilities. Following on from this argument is the fear that providing information to patients about the seriousness of their illnesses might well be harmful to them and that it is often best for the doctor to protect patients from the possible emotional consequences of such disclosure.

PROFESSIONAL AUTHORITY

An opposing view (Freidson 1970) is that the difference between the medical interview and other information-giving circumstances is not due to any emotional difficulty within the consultation but more an inevitable result of doctors' desire to retain their high status within society. This analysis suggests a much less altruistic reason for withholding information. If the difference in social standing between doctor and patient is something that the profession desperately wishes to preserve, in part this can be achieved by limiting the provision of information to the lay population. Mystification of the doctor's and devaluation of the patient's knowledge might be said to be more powerful driving forces than the higher motive of creating informed and autonomous patients. Maintaining clear water between professional and client necessitates a degree of ownership of information by the doctor. The use of Latin terms can be seen as one part of this complicated process of obfuscation – the patient presents with a sore throat, the doctor advises that it is acute pharyngitis. Of course, this impressive title is simply a translation of the patient's words into an unshared medical language (Bouhris *et al*. 1989).

The perceived 'competence gap', the emotional difficulties of the doctor–patient relationship and the need to preserve professional authority may then have predisposed physicians to withhold information and patients to remain passive bystanders in the explanation and planning phase of the interview.

Why has modern research been misinterpreted as confirming the traditional stereotype of information giving?

Tuckett *et al*. (1985) have argued that the medical profession has incorrectly interpreted some of the results of research into information giving so as to confirm its own traditional prejudices.

EARLY STUDIES OF RECALL OF INFORMATION

In earlier studies, patients' recall of information was shown to be poor. Ley (1988) quoted figures of around 60% in hospital settings from various authors, with better recall in repeat rather than new interviews. In general practice, Ley found 50% and 56% recall respectively. Bertakis (1977) showed 62% recall in first attenders and Hulka (1979), mainly with repeat consultations, showed higher levels of 67% for diabetics and pregnant mothers and 88% for mothers whose infants were ill.

Ley also demonstrated a relationship between the amount of information presented and the amount of information recalled. His research showed that in laboratory experiments, the more items of information given, the greater the proportion forgotten. He was able to confirm this finding in the clinical situation of hospital out-patients although not in general practice. This research has been widely quoted as evidence that:

- 'patients recall very little of what you tell them'
- 'the more you tell them the less they remember'

and the almost inevitable conclusion

- 'it's therefore not worth telling them very much in the first place'.

But are these conclusions correct? Even if only 50% of information is remembered, does that mean that it is not worth giving information at all or does it suggest that we should look at ways of improving that figure?

MORE RECENT STUDIES

More recent research suggests that patients actually recall much more than had previously been described. Tuckett *et al*. (1985), using a different methodology which looked more closely at what was being recalled and specifically analysed key points rather than every piece of information given by the doctor, showed that only 10% of patients in a study in primary care failed to remember all of the key points that they had been told.

Ley, in fact, never meant to imply that we should not strive to give patients information (Ley 1988). Commenting on his work on the relationship between the amount of information presented and the amount of information recalled, he makes the following point: 'Note that it is the proportion forgotten that increases and this is quite compatible with patients given more information about their disease knowing more about their condition than those given less. The finding is not an argument for providing patients with less information.' Although the proportion of the total remembered goes down, the absolute amount remembered still goes up.

CONFIRMATION OF PREJUDICES

Tuckett has written eloquently of how these misconceptions concerning Ley's findings have confirmed the medical profession's traditional views and been accepted as standard teaching (Tuckett *et al.* 1985). Those aspects of Ley's works that fit well into the traditional model have reached prominence – those that do not have been discarded. In the past, students have been told that patients will not remember most of what they are told and that they should keep it simple. They have been taught not to be overambitious in information giving and that 'only when the number of statements is limited to two is recall good' (Horder *et al.* 1972). Doctors have seized on Ley's findings to justify their view that there is little scope for more than basic information giving. Yet, as mentioned above, these were not Ley's own conclusions. His view was that doctors should use strategies to improve the amount of information given to patients and the total of that information which their patients can then recall and understand. He wished doctors to give more, clearer and better ordered information and for patients to become better informed.

What recent trends have influenced medical information giving?

CHANGES IN SOCIETY

Recent decades have brought many changes in society and the breaking down of a multitude of class and social barriers. Moves towards freedom of speech, sexual and racial equality and freedom of information have changed society irrevocably. As educational standards and personal wealth have increased, expectations have followed suit and demands have escalated on many services, including health. Changes away from just curative medicine towards prevention of illness and maintenance of health have led to an increased awareness of health issues in the population. The mushrooming of articles and programmes in the written and broadcast media has led to much greater availability of information about health and disease, and the emergence of consumer and patient support groups has changed the influence of the patient on the consultation. Society has not stood still and nor has the doctor–patient relationship; the public routinely questions both the knowledge and motivation of doctors and no longer demonstrates a blind faith in the profession. Patients do not now accept the concept of an unbridgeable competence gap.

CHANGES IN MEDICINE

While patients may well adopt a dependent role with very serious illness and be only too grateful for the doctor to take charge, most consultations in modern, Western medical practice are not about life-threatening illness. Furthermore, chronic care and prevention are playing increasingly larger roles. As a result, anxiety levels and consequent blocks to communication are reduced; patients feel that they can cope with being fully informed and involved in their care.

PATIENT AUTONOMY

Patient autonomy has become a central tenet of medical ethics and the paternalistic relationship between doctor and patient is increasingly viewed as anachronistic. As we shall see later, there is a danger of too large a shift towards a consumerist relationship; a collaborative and mutual approach has been suggested as a more appropriate path forwards.

Doctors have seen these changes gradually reflected in their working practices. Patients far more frequently come for information about preventative measures such as hormone replacement therapy with the expectation that they themselves will make an informed decision based on the arguments put before them – in the past the doctor would simply have made a recommendation and expected the patient to follow. Ward rounds less frequently consist of discussions at the end of the bed about patients who are considered to have no thoughts or feelings or involvement in the process of their own medical care. Perhaps the biggest change has been in the area of withholding information about serious illness or bad news. Not long ago, it was the norm to withhold news of conditions such as cancer from patients on the basis that the information might harm the patient. Physicians shielded their patients from information that they might not be able to cope with. It was the physician's responsibility to decide whether to favour discretion and complicity with relatives over the duty to tell the truth. Now, the pendulum has swung to the patient's right to information, for the physician to provide opportunities to inform patients sensitively about their disease and withhold that information only if the patient gives out signals that they would prefer not to know (Buckman 1994).

What is the research evidence to suggest that giving more information is helpful?

Patients wish to receive more information than they are routinely given. But can we demonstrate that this provision of information actually affects the outcome of their health care?

There is much evidence to confirm the value of information giving. In a meta-analysis of the influence of the various 'provider behaviours' that might make a difference in medical encounters, Hall et al. (1988) searched the literature from 1966 to 1985 and discovered 41 independent studies where communication variables by the health professional were related to improvements in satisfaction, recall or compliance. Having grouped the possible variables into six overall categories, their conclusion was that, of all the categories, the amount of information imparted by physicians was the most dramatic predictor of patient satisfaction, compliance, recall and understanding. This positive relationship between patient satisfaction and the amount of information given is a highly consistent finding in the communication literature (e.g. Bertakis 1977; Stiles *et al.* 1979; Deyo and Diehl 1986).

Many studies link the provision of information to substantial benefits in health outcomes such as symptom reduction and physiological status (Kaplan *et al.* 1989; Stewart 1995). Egbert *et al.* (1964) showed that pre-operative education from an anaesthetist about post-operative pain control led not only to less use of analgesia but to shorter hospital stays. Mumford *et al.* (1982) reviewed many similar findings of information giving or psychological intervention speeding recovery and improving outcome in patients post-surgery or post-myocardial infarction.

Do all patients want more information?

But do all patients want more information and, if not, how can doctors individualize their information giving to match their patients' needs?

In Pinder's (1990) study of information giving to patients with Parkinson's disease, doctors adopted a set style with all patients despite individual patients varying greatly in the amount of information that they wished to know. Most patients were keen to hear more information about their illness and medication, but not all. Many studies have shown that patients can be divided into seekers (80%) and avoiders (20%) concerning information, with seekers coping better with more information and avoiders with less (Miller and Mangan 1983; Deber 1994). Steptoe *et al.* (1991) showed that information avoiders report a better understanding and satisfaction with doctor–patient communication than seekers but paradoxically have a worse understanding; seekers on the other hand are less satisfied with communication and would like even more information despite having already gained a better understanding. Tuckett *et al.* (1985) found that 19% of patients did not ask questions of their doctors because they were not interested in knowing about medical matters. Broyles *et al.* (1992) showed that only half of mothers of newborn babies at risk of respiratory failure, when presented with brief information about mechanical ventilation and then asked if they wished to have further detailed information, requested more.

While most patients do want their doctors to provide more information, a minority would like less. But it is not at all easy to predict which patient is in which group. For instance, as Waitzkin (1985) said, 'Research has clearly shown that the commonly expressed assumption that working-class patients do not want a full explanation of their illness seems to derive from the hesitancy of patients to ask questions rather than from any actual disinterest in information'. Barsevich and Johnson (1990) showed that there was only a moderate relationship between the information wishes of women undergoing colposcopy and their information-seeking behaviour. One of the key challenges in information giving is how to tailor the amount of information to the needs of the individual patient without making false assumptions. In the past, we have tended to withhold information from all to protect the few who would rather not know. The new challenge is how to inform the majority while being sensitive to the needs of the minority.

What skills can learners use to help gauge the correct amount and type of information to give to each individual patient?

CHUNKING AND CHECKING

Chunking and checking is of central importance throughout the explanation and planning phase of the interview, not only for gauging the correct amount of information to give but also as an aid to accurate recall and to achieving a shared understanding. We explore this vital skill in the next section of this chapter.

ASSESSING THE PATIENT'S STARTING POINT

One key interactive approach to giving information to patients involves assessing the patient's prior knowledge. How can you determine at what level to pitch information unless you take active steps to find out the patient's starting point? How can you assess the degree to which your view of the problem differs from that of the patient and the approach that you will need to take to achieve mutual understanding unless you discover early on the patient's understanding of their problem?

Explaining a new diagnosis of diabetes to either a university lecturer or a manual labourer is apparently not the same task, with potentially very different levels of understanding and different capabilities of processing information. But making this assumption without directly asking for the patient's prior knowledge is highly dangerous. The lecturer in astronomy may have a poor understanding of diabetes and know it only as a possibly disastrous cause of blindness and a threat to his vocation. The labourer may have grown up with parents with diabetes and have a high level of understanding of the condition. It would therefore be helpful before proceeding too far into a detailed explanation to ask:

'I don't know how much you know about diabetes already?'
'Well, I know something about it – my best friend at college had it.'
'It would be helpful for me to understand a little of what you already know so that I can try to fill in any gaps for you.'

Similarly, it is important to discover each individual patient's overall desire for information. As we have already seen, while most patients wish their doctors to provide more information, a significant minority prefer less. How can we discover if a particular patient is a seeker or avoider of information? Chunking and checking and asking for patients' questions are indirect approaches to assessing our patients' overall information needs. A more direct approach is to ask the patient early on in the process:

'There's a lot more information that I'd be happy to share with you about Parkinson's disease and the drugs we use to treat it. Some patients like to know a lot about these things and some prefer to keep it to a minimum – how much information would you yourself like?'

Remember that a patient's preference and need for information may change over time and from situation to situation. For instance, a terminally ill patient may move from a position of avoidance and denial towards acceptance and more open discussion as he comes to terms with his illness. We need to be aware of this possibility and not assume that the answer to the above question will remain constant for any one individual.

ASKING PATIENTS WHAT OTHER INFORMATION WOULD BE HELPFUL

As we have seen, doctors often misconstrue the types of information that the patient wishes to receive. They often do not address the 'what has happened, why has it happened, why to me, why now, what would happen if nothing was done about it' questions that patients would like answering in preference to information about treatment (Helman 1978). It is difficult to guess each patient's individual needs and asking directly is an obvious way to prevent the omission of important information:

'Are there any other questions you'd like me to answer or any points I haven't covered?'

GIVING EXPLANATION AT APPROPRIATE TIMES

A common difficulty in consultations arises from giving advice, information or reassurance prematurely. For instance, during the information-gathering phase, a mother of an asthmatic child says:

'Sophie's really sick with this cold – could she have some antibiotics?'
and you answer:
'I'm sure the answer isn't antibiotics. Her cold will have triggered off her asthma – it's not that she has infection on her chest. What we really need to do is treat the asthma.' You deliver your standard lecture. You then take more history and find that Sophie has been hot and sick in the night. Examination reveals unilateral signs. You start backtracking and feel you have lost the mother's confidence:
'Ah, despite what I said there is a problem here that needs antibiotics.'
Instead, you could simply acknowledge the mother's question and deal with it later after you have all the facts at your disposal:
'That's a very good question. Would you mind if I put that on hold just for a second and come back to it after I've examined Sophie – then I'll be able to give you a much better answer.'

Then after you have explained your findings:

'Coming back to your question – there clearly is a problem with her chest today that needs antibiotics. Are you happy gauging when it is the asthma itself that's worse and when she might have a chest infection?'
'Yes, I think so but it's not always easy.'
'Well, on most occasions, it's just that a cold triggers asthma without the infection going on to the chest …'

SECTION 2: AIDING ACCURATE RECALL AND UNDERSTANDING

Another important area in explanation and planning is how to give information that can be more easily remembered and understood.

Ley's research into patient recall

In the 1970s and 1980s, Ley (1988) undertook comprehensive research to establish which communication skills could improve patients' recall of information. His work was initially based on experiments in the psychology laboratory. He later transposed his research into clinical settings: doctors in both hospital and general practice were taught various techniques to see if earlier laboratory findings could be reproduced in the consulting room. The following is our interpretation of Ley's findings.

CATEGORIZATION AND SIGNPOSTING

In this technique, the clinician forewarns the patient about which categories of information are to be provided and then presents the information category by category:

'There are three important things I want to explain. First I want to tell you what I think is wrong, second, what tests we should do and third, what the treatment might be. First, I think you have ...'

Ley demonstrated that recall was higher using this method in both laboratory and clinical experiments, with typical increases in recall rates from 50% to 64%.

There are two processes at work here. The first is the organization of information giving. Categorization allows doctors to divide information into discrete sections which they can then present in a logical sequence. The second is making that categorization explicit to the patient. This is a further example of signposting, a technique that we introduced in Chapter 3. Signposting is the process of explaining to the patient where the interview might go next and why. Providing an overt structure to the consultation reduces uncertainty and anxiety which can otherwise block effective communication and reduce recall and understanding.

LABELLING IMPORTANT INFORMATION

Ley places much emphasis in his writings on the primacy effect, that people remember best what they are told first. He demonstrated in laboratory experiments that medical facts given to volunteers early in a sequence of information were recalled more than those given later. He then proceeded to a clinical setting. Ley had previously shown that patients recalled information about diagnosis better than information about instructions and advice since patients considered information about diagnosis to be more important than information about treatment. People recall better what they think is most important. To see if recall of instructions and advice could be improved he used the out-patient setting to give information in varying orders. Patients who were given information about treatment first remembered 86% of this information compared to 50% in patients who were given the information later. Interestingly, there was no improvement in the amount of information retained overall – as recall of instructions and advice increased, so recall of diagnosis declined.

While the primacy effect is clearly of importance in information giving, we do have some reservations about Ley's conclusion that we should present 'important' information first. Ley's work suggests that to increase compliance we should give information about treatment and advice before diagnosis and rationale. This view is based on the premise that patients remember treatment issues less well and that compliance with treatment plans will suffer if recall is not maximized. But total recall remains unchanged and in Ley's study recall of diagnosis and rationale diminished. Although remembering treatment plans is a necessary condition for compliance, will this approach actually achieve increased adherence to plans in practice or are there other factors involved? Ley has already said that patients view diagnostic statements as more important than instruction and advice, so does it not seem likely that reducing patients' understanding about their diagnosis will have deleterious effects on their compliance? What if the patient remembers exactly what the doctor said about treatment but has no intention of complying because he has little understanding of his condition or commitment to the doctor's views:

'He told me to take this steroid inhaler twice a day all the time but I'm fine now so I don't need to take anything.'

Clearly, recall is not everything. And who is to say what is the most 'important' information? What the patient and doctor think is important might be completely different. Ley's approach here is doctor-centred in that it is the doctor who decides what is the most important information for the patient to understand. It runs contrary to the work of Tuckett *et al.* (1985), presented in the next section, where the importance of discovering and addressing each patient's very individual information needs is emphasized.

One further message of value here is Ley's finding that it might help if the physician labels certain pieces of information as important to raise the patient's awareness of his perception. This is another example of signposting:

'It is very important that you remember this ...'

CHUNKING AND CHECKING

We would argue that the key issue here is not so much about ordering information but about avoiding giving a large amount of information all at once. A long monologue will produce a strong primacy effect – the patient is still thinking about the first point as the next three are being presented and is distracted from listening to later pieces of information. If the aim is to increase recall, understanding and commitment to plans, we suggest reducing the likelihood of a primacy effect occurring in the first place.

This can be achieved by giving information in small pieces, pausing and checking for understanding before proceeding and being guided by the patient's reactions to see what information is required next. Only then is it likely that patients will both recall and understand; as they assimilate each section of information, they will become ready for the next. This technique is also a vital component of assessing the patient's overall information needs; if information is given in small chunks and the patient given ample opportunity to contribute, the doctor will receive clear signals about the amount and type of information still required by the patient.

REPETITION

There are two elements to repetition that can make a considerable difference to patient recall:

1 repetition of important points by the doctor
2 restatement of information by the patient.

Repetition by the doctor of important points has been shown to be of value in assisting recall in laboratory conditions (Ley) and in the consulting room (Kupst *et al.* 1975). Kupst showed immediate recall to be 76% for single presentation and 90% after physician repetition.

Patient restatement is a highly effective technique. Here the doctor checks the patient's understanding of information given by asking her to restate in her own words what she has understood. The doctor then clarifies as necessary. In Kupst's work, patient restatement achieved 91% immediate recall, which matched physician repetition. However, for recall at one month, patient restatement with feedback was shown to be the most effective method.

Bertakis (1977) undertook a study to evaluate the usefulness of patient restatement and physician clarification. When family practice residents were trained in this technique, patients were more satisfied and showed an increase from 61% to 83% in retention of information.

LANGUAGE

We have seen that the use of jargon is a major problem in communication and that patients rarely ask for clarification for fear of appearing ignorant. It is not just technical language that is the problem (Hadlow and Pitts 1991) as even simple everyday words in a medical context can be ambiguous. Mazzullo *et al.* (1974) showed that 52% of people thought that a medication prescribed 'for fluid retention' would cause fluid retention. Ley therefore recommends simplification of information to aid recall and understanding. This can be achieved by:

- the reduction in use of jargon
- the explanation of jargon when used
- the use of shorter words
- the use of shorter sentences.

MAKING EXPLANATIONS OR ADVICE SPECIFIC ENOUGH FOR THE PATIENT TO UNDERSTAND OR ACT UPON

Ley quotes Bradshaw *et al.* (1975) to demonstrate that specific statements are more easily recalled than general statements – obese women given dietary advice remembered 16% of general and 51% of specific statements.

Making advice more specific clearly makes sense in certain situations such as explaining to patients how to take pills. But we have reservations about promulgating this method in all circumstances of information giving; there is a danger that giving specific advice can become confused with being inappropriately dogmatic.

As we shall see later, there is much evidence to favour a collaborative model of explanation and planning where patients are involved in choices and doctors offer options and suggestions rather than directives. Adherence to plans has been shown to be improved when doctors actively seek patients' reactions to suggestions and engage in appropriate negotiations. Ley suggests that telling a patient to lose 30 pounds will lead to better recall than just telling the patient to lose weight. But will this produce better compliance? What if all the patient remembers is:

'30 pounds! I've never been that weight in my life – no way!'

There is a third approach. Make suggestions, elicit reactions and negotiate. Then, at the end of that process, clarify specifically what the agreed plan involves. How to use 'being specific' therefore depends upon the complexity of the task. In simple instructions, being specific is relatively easy. But in complex areas such as health promotion or preventive medicine, it is pointless engineering excellent recall without motivation. Being specific needs to be balanced by the skills of negotiation and motivational interviewing.

USING VISUAL METHODS OF CONVEYING INFORMATION

Many studies have shown that the use of diagrams, models, written information and instructions can improve patient knowledge and compliance; there is considerable literature on the effective design of printed material to improve patient use, understanding and recall which is well summarized in Ley (1988).

A summary of the skills that can help patients remember and understand doctors' explanations is given in Box 5.1 (p. 93).

SECTION 3: ACHIEVING A SHARED UNDERSTANDING: INCORPORATING THE PATIENT'S PERSPECTIVE

In the above analysis of Ley's (1988) work, we have looked in detail at the skills that can be employed to improve patients' recall of information. This approach is concerned primarily with the recall of information that doctors consider to be important. But as we have already seen from the work of Kindelan and Kent (1987) and indeed from Ley's own analysis, what the patient and doctor think is important is not always the same. So just looking at what doctors think their patients should be told and discovering the best ways to give that information is only half the story: what about the information needs from the patient's perspective (Grol *et al.* 1991)?

Asking this question does not negate Ley's findings; he presents important skills that doctors can use to make information giving clearer and that can lead to better patient recall. But a further analysis is needed of how to match information giving to patients' perceived needs. How do you provide explanations that relate to the patient's perspective of the problem? How do you discover the patient's thoughts about the information that you have given? How do you achieve a shared understanding with your patients?

Tuckett and colleagues' research into patient understanding

Tuckett *et al.*'s research, described in their book *Meetings between experts: an approach to sharing ideas in the medical consultation* (1985), is central to our understanding of a shared approach to information giving. Their use of a different methodological approach has greatly extended our understanding and has challenged our previous perceptions.

TUCKETT ET AL.'S METHODOLOGY

Tuckett *et al.* studied 1302 consultations conducted by 16 doctors in British general practice, in considerable depth, setting out with the following principles in mind:

- *Not all information is of equal importance*. Previous work had assessed information giving by counting how many of the total number of statements made by the doctor were remembered by the patient. But perhaps some information is more important than other information. Does it matter that patients forget a certain proportion of information given if they remember the most important points? Does it help if patients remember more statements if this is not the information they really need to understand their problem? We need to consider what information has been imparted as well as how much.
- *Recall does not necessarily imply understanding or commitment*. Just improving recall will not necessarily lead to better health outcomes. What if the patient can recall what the doctor said but it appears to make no sense? We have to look beyond recall to understanding; although recall is important, it is not by itself a satisfactory endpoint in information-giving research.
- *Information giving needs to be looked at from the patient's perspective as well as the doctor's*. The problem of information giving is not simply about how doctors can give information that they wish to impart. It is also about how patients can discover the information they themselves would like and how doctors can assist in that process.

Tuckett *et al.*'s first step in exploring these issues was to devise a framework of information giving. If some information is more important than others, a theoretical framework is required to subdivide information so that analysis can go further than just counting the total number of statements made or the total time spent in information giving. This framework was devised by looking at information giving from both the doctor's and the patient's perspective. Ideas were taken from the disease-based approach of traditional medicine and married with the illness perspective of more contemporary theories of medical communication and, in particular, with the work of social anthropologists such as Helman (1978) ('what has happened, why has it happened, why to me, why now, what would happen if nothing was done about it, what should I do about it?'):

- **the diagnostic significance of a problem:** diagnosis (what it is), aetiology (what caused it), severity (whether serious, life-threatening, self-limiting), prognosis (likely to recur, expected outcome)
- **the appropriate treatment action:** what investigations and treatments are recommended, their value and purpose, risks and benefits, how they are carried out
- **the appropriate preventive measures:** their value and purpose, how they relate to the cause and how to carry them out
- **the implications:** the wider social and emotional consequences of the problem or the proposed treatment (the social consequences to the patient, their psychological reaction and how they can be helped to cope).

For each of these areas, information giving was further considered in two segments:

1 the doctor's view (stating the view – clarifying, making plain)
2 the doctor's rationale (justification and support).

Next, Tuckett's team devised a method of deciding what were the 'key' points made by the doctor. This enabled the subsequent analysis of patient recall to be examined in relation not to all possible statements made by the doctor but only to those important statements necessary for the patient to make sense of their illness and treatment.

Their third step was to go further than patient recall as a measure of outcome and into the more significant realm of patient understanding and commitment. They therefore looked at the following three outcome measures:

1 **patient recall**
2 **patient understanding:** did the patient make correct sense of what they were told?
3 **patient commitment:** did the patient agree with the doctor's key ideas and were these ideas in conflict with their own explanatory models?

The fourth and last step taken by Tuckett *et al.* was to look at 'how' doctors gave information. Firstly, they examined Ley's concept of clarity in information giving. What influence did doctors' abilities to use Ley's suggestions have on patient recall, understanding and commitment? Secondly, they looked at a totally different perspective, mutual sharing by exchange of views which is very similar to the disease–illness model, the all-important theoretical model that we explored in Chapter 3. Does understanding the patient's belief systems and taking into account the patient's own perspective of their illness help information giving? They therefore looked at:

- clarity
  - explicit categorization
  - grammatical statements
  - coherence of phraseology
  - avoidance of jargon
  - avoidance of unexplained assumptions
  - pace and audibility
- mutual sharing by exchange of views
  - doctors' efforts to encourage patients to volunteer and elaborate on their ideas
  - doctors' responses to any evidence of patients having ideas
  - the extent to which doctors' reasoning was directly related to patients' ideas
  - the extent to which doctors checked for patient understanding.

WHAT DOES TUCKETT AND COLLEAGUES' RESEARCH SHOW ABOUT THE INFORMATION GIVEN BY DOCTORS?

- As expected, doctors' information giving placed far more emphasis on diagnostic significance and treatment action than preventive action or implications.
- On only a small percentage of occasions were doctors' views presented clearly.
- On only 50% of occasions were rationales included to substantiate doctors' views.
- Even when rationales were given, they were mostly lacking in content and clarity.
- Doctors almost never related their explanations to patients' views or beliefs – in only 12 out of 405 consultations were doctors' explanations related to their patients' beliefs at all.

- In only 6% of consultations were patients' ideas and explanatory beliefs elicited in the first place.
- Even when patients volunteered their ideas either as hinted cues or as spontaneous outright statements, doctors still only asked patients to elaborate on their ideas in 7% of consultations.
- Not only were patients not asked to elaborate on their ideas, doctors often evaded them, interrupted them or deliberately inhibited their expression.
- In only 7% of consultations did doctors in any way check their patients' understanding of what had been said.

In summary, Tuckett *et al.*'s research showed that doctors rarely exhibited the organizational and linguistic skills to make their efforts at communication clear to patients. They also showed little interest in their patients' theories, hypotheses or understanding. Therefore, in relation to both models of 'how' to give information (Ley's and the disease–illness model) doctors would not be expected to be particularly effective in their efforts at information giving!

WHAT DOES TUCKETT AND COLLEAGUES' RESEARCH SHOW ABOUT THE INFLUENCE PATIENTS CAN HAVE ON THEIR DOCTORS' INFORMATION GIVING?

Do patients attempt to influence their doctors' information giving and do they do it overtly or covertly? To assess how often patients tried to play an active role in this part of the consultation, Tuckett *et al.* examined the following strategies that could be used by patients to influence the information obtained from their doctors:

- indicating their own explanatory models
- seeking clarification of a doctor's views and instructions
- asking for a doctor's reasons and rationales
- expressing doubts.

They could do this:

- overtly
- covertly.

A remarkably high level of participation was demonstrated. In fact, 85% of patients engaged in at least one of the four activities. However, this participation was mostly performed in a covert way, utilizing hints and vague questions rather than overtly, with clear statements or questions. This fits in well with other work showing that the proportion of patients asking overt questions is small (Svarstad 1974; Roter 1977; Stimson and Webb 1975; Beisecker and Beisecker 1990).

What effects did patients' participation have on doctors' information giving? When patients did contribute overtly, they were more likely to receive more information. Covert participation led to a much smaller effect. Svarstad (1974), Boreham and Gibson (1978) and Roter (1977) have also shown that when patients ask questions overtly, doctors provide answers and patients obtain more detailed explanations.

So, patients can exert considerable control over how their physicians behave and are wise to ask questions openly rather than covertly if they wish to receive more information. However, there is a potentially less desirable outcome. Where doctors did not respond positively to patients asking them for their rationale or expressing doubts, patients were more likely to experience a consultation characterized by evasive attitudes and behaviour from the doctor and an increase in tension. Roter (1977) also found that more patient questioning led to increased doctor anxiety and anger. As we shall see later, this apparently negative outcome may in fact enhance communication.

Do patients feel they would like to ask their doctors questions, and if so, why don't they do so overtly? In Tuckett *et al.*'s research, 76% of the patients said afterwards that they had specific doubts or questions during the interview that they did not mention to the doctor. Why do patients hold back from asking questions? And why, when they do pluck up courage, do they often ask questions covertly and provide only indirect cues to their information needs? Patients in the study gave the following reasons for their behaviour:

- not up to them to ask questions, express doubts or behave as if their view was important (36%)
- afraid of being less well thought of by the doctor (22%)
- frightened of a negative reaction from the doctor (14%)
- too flustered or hurried to ask coherently (27%)
- doubted that the doctor could tell them any more at the moment (22%)
- forgot or waiting until next time to ask when they would be more certain of what they thought was reasonable to ask (36%)
- fear of the truth (9%).

Only 19% of patients who exhibited gaps in their knowledge at interview said that they did not ask questions because they were not interested in the answer.

WHAT ARE THE COMBINED EFFECTS OF PATIENTS' AND DOCTORS' APPROACHES TO PATIENT INVOLVEMENT IN INFORMATION GIVING?

Tying together Tuckett *et al.*'s results of both patients' and doctors' behaviour in the consultation leads to some depressing conclusions. Both parties appeared to adopt the roles predicted by the traditional view of the doctor–patient relationship. Patients felt that it was not relevant for them to understand or up to them to ask questions. They were afraid of the doctors' reactions to questions that they might ask. Eighty-five per cent of patients attempted to contribute their ideas or ask questions or express doubts but the majority employed hints and vague questions rather than overt questions. Doctors were poor at picking up on such cues or covert messages, did not encourage and even actively discouraged patients from expressing their ideas and often responded with increased tension when ideas were ventured or questions were asked. Therefore, doctors' behaviour and patients' perceptions together act to confirm a passive role for the patient in which shared understanding is unlikely to occur.

The tradition of the doctor controlling information appears to be very strong; patients adopt a passive role and are assumed to be uninterested by doctors who take the initiative. Unfortunately, doctors' and patients' behaviours are self-perpetuating; past experiences of patients and physicians tend to reinforce the attitudes of authority and deference that overshadow the doctor–patient relationship.

CAN DOCTORS AND PATIENTS MORE POSITIVELY INFLUENCE EACH OTHER TOWARDS A SHARED UNDERSTANDING IN INFORMATION GIVING?

We have already seen that the more active patients are in the consultation, the more likely they are to obtain the information they would like. There is also no doubt that doctors, if they wish, can influence patients and enable them to take a more active role. Svarstad (1974) showed that doctors who avoided certain inhibiting behaviours enabled their patients to ask more questions. Inhibiting conditions included: clock-watching, use of jargon, mumbling incomprehensibly, interrupting, ignoring patients' comments, unfriendliness and ending consultations precipitately. Doctors appeared to be able to vary their behaviour according to circumstances and used communication-limiting strategies much more when they were under pressure of time. So both doctors and patients can influence the degree of sharing that occurs in the consultation.

DOES TUCKETT ET AL.'S RESEARCH ABOUT RECALL FIT IN WITH PREVIOUS WORK?

One very important finding of Tuckett *et al.*'s work is that patients recalled far more information than previous studies had intimated. Tuckett *et al.* found that only 10% of information was forgotten as opposed to 30–50% in studies such as those of Ley. As doctors had in the past used patients' poor recall to justify giving only limited information to patients, this new finding was of extreme importance. What could be the reason for this significant difference?

Although it is possible that differences in the settings in which the interviews studied took place may have been responsible, by far the most likely cause is the different methodology for assessing recall used by Tuckett's team. Firstly, they assessed only whether patients remembered the 'key' points made by the doctor in each of the four categories of their framework. This is very different from seeing how many statements were remembered of all the things said by the doctor. Secondly, while previous work had used the method of free recall, whereby interviewers asked a general question such as 'What did the doctor say to you about the reasons for seeing him?' and were then not allowed to probe any further, Tuckett *et al.* used the approach of probed recall, where interviewers used a standardized interview but were allowed to ask about the patient's meaning and clarify answers.

WAS CORRECT SENSE MADE OF THE EXPLANATIONS?

Ninety per cent of the key points of information provided by their doctors were remembered. But was it understood? Tuckett *et al.* compared patients' understanding of the information that they had received with their doctors' actual meaning, as judged by third-party assessment. Again, high levels of comprehension were found: 73% of patients made correct sense of the key points they had been told.

Tuckett *et al.* then looked at the effect that the two different concepts of 'how' to give information, clarity and mutual sharing by exchange of views, had on patient understanding. Surprisingly, no relationship was found at all between the clarity of explanation given by the doctor and whether correct sense was made of the doctor's comments by the patient! Clarity appeared to make little difference to understanding.

Attempts to correlate the value of mutual sharing to patient understanding did, however, produce evidence of a relationship. Consultations in which the doctor inhibited or evaded their patients' ideas were more likely to result in a failure of recall and understanding.

Understanding dropped from 40% to 29%. This suggests that paying attention to the patients' explanatory framework does increase understanding. It was not possible to assess other aspects of mutual sharing because doctors so rarely demonstrated the appropriate skills required. Patients' understanding was so rarely checked and clarified by the doctor, patients' ideas and beliefs were so infrequently actively discovered and the rationales given were so rarely related to patients' explanatory beliefs that their effect on understanding could not be ascertained!

To try to discover further information about the importance of a mutual exchange of views, Tuckett *et al.* undertook a qualitative analysis of a small sample of the consultations. Further examination of the recorded consultations and post-consultation interviews showed that patients had particular problems with recall and making sense of information presented by the doctor when there was a mismatch with the patient's own explanatory framework. The key to the problem of understanding appeared to be the detailed ideas that the patient brought to bear on the explanation of the doctor – if there was a match with the doctor's explanation, good understanding ensued, even if the explanation by the doctor had been unclear or sparse. However, if there was a mismatch in the doctor's and the patient's explanatory frameworks, understanding was likely to suffer. It is, not surprisingly, more difficult to assimilate information which is unfamiliar, unexpected or threatening; then, the ambiguous and disorganized information giving of doctors is likely to be particularly unhelpful.

Poor information giving clearly leads to considerable scope for misunderstanding. If the doctor's and patient's views are divergent, the patient could arrive at a very different version of what the doctor was trying to say without either party realizing. If the doctor has not discovered the patient's views, nor conveyed explicitly that his views differ nor checked the patient's understanding after giving the information, the patient may well misinterpret information or even assume incorrectly that the doctor is confirming the patient's views. In contrast, if views are very close, doctors will escape the consequences of disorganization and ambiguity as there is already a congruity of views and much less likelihood of misunderstanding.

WERE PATIENTS COMMITTED TO THE DOCTOR'S VIEW?

The overwhelming majority (75%) of patients who had remembered and made sense of information that they were given were also committed to the doctor's views. Again, consultations in which the doctor inhibited or evaded their patient's ideas were more likely to result in lack of commitment to the doctor's views.

The qualitative analysis showed a major difference between those patients that were committed to a doctor's view and those that were not. Those committed usually expected what they heard and already agreed with it. However, if the patient started out with views divergent from the doctor, the consultations appeared to do little to change them. Patients rejected the doctors' views in favour of their own. As doctors rarely paid attention to patients' ideas, they remained uninformed about their patients' thinking and could not direct their explanations precisely to it. Tuckett *et al.* firmly believe that without establishing what ideas the patient has, there is no possibility of a mutual exchange of views, and without this there is little likelihood of increasing commitment.

As we have said, many patients expressed doubts or asked the doctor for further explanations of his rationale. Tuckett *et al.* showed that patients who demonstrated evidence of questioning their doctor in these ways were more likely not to be committed to the doctor's view by the end of the consultation. Patients, it seems, are keen to warn us of the need to take their views and thinking seriously and yet, by and large, we ignore their efforts to engineer a mutual exploration of ideas.

WHAT ARE TUCKETT ET AL.'S MAIN CONCLUSIONS?

Tuckett *et al.* have therefore shown that consultations go wrong where there is an incongruity between the patient's and the doctor's explanatory frameworks. The lack of doctors' efforts to treat patients' views and theories as important and to find some way of relating medical models to patients' ideas when they are in opposition is, in their view, the main cause of unsuccessful outcomes. Doctors need to explore their patients' views and beliefs and subsequently incorporate them into their explanations. They conclude that there is a need for two concerted approaches to encourage success in our goals of patient recall, understanding and commitment:

1 clarity – so that the patient can understand what is said and comprehend if there is a difference between the doctor's and their own beliefs
2 exploration of the patient's beliefs and ideas together with checking the patient's interpretation and reaction to information given. The doctor needs to be willing to explore the differences in viewpoint and negotiate a shared explanatory model.

Tuckett *et al.* suggest that the traditional view of the doctor–patient relationship has devalued the patient's contribution and prevented an exchange of views. We need to change our approach to explanation and planning to enable a 'meeting between experts', an explicit sharing of explanatory models between two parties with different expertise, one of the medical world and one of the unique experience of the individual. Unfortunately, Tuckett *et al.* were not able to take the last step to completely prove this hypothesis. Although it is clear from their work that differences in explanatory framework lead to poorer understanding and commitment, they could not produce direct evidence to prove the efficacy of the measures that they proposed to combat this problem. So few consultations demonstrated an active search for patients' ideas or included explanations that were related to patients' explanatory frameworks that a statistical analysis proved impossible. We are still left with the partially unanswered question: if we do elicit our patients' conflicting ideas, take them into account and explain our findings in relation to them, will we improve our patients' understanding and commitment?

Other work to support shared understanding

Tuckett *et al.*'s concept of an 'explicit sharing of explanatory models' fits very well with the disease–illness model, as discussed in Chapter 3. There we advocated a three-stage plan for discovering patients' beliefs:

1 identification
2 acceptance
3 explanation

in which integrating doctors' and patients' understanding of problems and reaching mutually understood common ground is the final aim. What additional evidence supports this approach?

Eisenthal and Lazare (1976) (see Chapter 3) demonstrated that if physicians in a psychiatric walk-in clinic discovered patients' expectations, patients were more likely to feel satisfied and to adhere to plans whether their requests were granted or not. In other words, the reason for discovering expectations is not just so that you can give patients what they want but so that you can base your negotiation on an open understanding of your respective positions. Eliciting expectations allows the physician to consider the relevance of the patient's position and to produce evidence for and against different approaches. It is not finding out whether the patient wants a CT scan and going along with their wishes that is important but finding out their expectations, explaining the doctor's position in relation to their views and reaching a negotiated plan acceptable to both parties.

Arborelius and Bremberg (1992), in a study in general practice, showed that in those consultations where both doctor and patient rated the interview positively, increased efforts were made to establish the patient's ideas and concerns and more time was spent on the tasks of shared understanding and involving the patient in their own management.

Maynard (1990) used a qualitative approach to investigate the importance of discovering patients' prior knowledge and feelings in the context of giving information to parents about their children's developmental disabilities. In this 'breaking bad news' scenario, Maynard identified that 'interactional alignment' was a critical factor in determining how parents accepted the diagnosis of developmental delay. If the news was given without discovering the parents' knowledge and feelings about their child's condition, there was a high likelihood of outright rejection of the diagnosis. When the clinician discovered the parents' understanding first, there was a much greater chance that the news could be delivered in such a way as to allow the parents to accept the diagnosis. Maynard therefore recommends an interactional style of giving difficult information where the doctor aligns himself with the patient and can anticipate problems before they arise. Once rejection of information has occurred, it is very difficult to redress the balance.

Maynard's work may go some way in helping doctors to overcome the problems that have been identified by others' research. A consistent finding in the literature (Starfield *et al.* 1981; Bass and Cohen 1982) is that lack of agreement at the end of the consultation about the nature of the problem or the need for follow-up leads to a reduction in improvement of patient symptoms. One way of improving the situation would perhaps be to adopt Maynard's approach of 'interactional alignment'.

Inui *et al.* (1976) looked at the effect of a single training session on compliance-aiding interviewing skills given to physicians working with patients with known hypertension in hospital out-patient clinics. Physicians were given one tutorial lasting up to two hours which demonstrated that:

- non-compliance was widespread in their patients
- there was a high probability that poor blood pressure control was indicative of poor compliance (90% relationship)
- physicians should discuss their patients' knowledge, attitudes and beliefs about their hypertension and its treatment rather than just search for complications of hypertension
- physicians should switch from being purely diagnosticians to being patient educators; they should link their patients' beliefs, attitudes and understanding to their explanations as doctors, share their rationale and help patients to overcome barriers to adherence.

The results of this study not only showed that trained doctors spent more time in considering their patients' ideas and in patient education than did control physicians, that patients' understanding of their condition improved and that compliance increased but also that there was better control of hypertension even six months after the tutorial! Here then is good physiological outcome evidence for the concept of shared understanding. Similar increases in compliance following a single training session on compliance-aiding interviewing skills have since also been obtained in the context of patients with otitis media attending paediatric outpatients (Maiman *et al.* 1988).

Kaplan *et al.* (1989), as we describe in more detail in the next section of this chapter, coached patients to voice their questions and concerns in the medical interview. They found that the subsequent change in patient behaviour not only produced a dramatic difference in what happened in the interview itself but also led to improved physiological outcomes in both diabetes and hypertension.

What skills can we recommend to help achieve a shared understanding between doctors and patients?

Examples of the skills in action are:

- **Relate explanations to patient's illness framework:** to previously elicited beliefs, concerns and expectations. *'You mentioned earlier that you were concerned that you might have angina ... I can see why you might have thought that but in fact I think it's more likely to be a muscular pain ... let me explain why ...'*
- **Provide opportunities and encourage patient to contribute:** to ask questions, seek clarification or express doubts; responds appropriately. *'What questions does that leave you with? Is there anything I haven't covered or explained?'*
- **Pick up verbal and non-verbal cues:** patient's need to contribute information or ask questions; information overload; distress. *'You seem unhappy about the possibility of having surgery ...'*
- **Elicit patient's beliefs, reactions and concerns:** re information given, terms used; acknowledge and address where necessary. *'I'm not sure how that news has left you feeling ...'*

SECTION 4: PLANNING – SHARED DECISION MAKING

Following on from explanation comes planning. Not only have there been major advances in concepts of information giving, there have also been considerable moves to change the medical profession's approach to planning and decision making. Increasingly, medical researchers, educators and patient groups have advocated models incorporating negotiation and mutual collaboration to address the substantial problem of non-adherence which threatens to undermine much of our current effort in diagnosis and treatment. What is the theoretical and research evidence behind these claims?

The theory behind the negotiating, collaborative approach

FOUR MODELS OF THE DOCTOR–PATIENT RELATIONSHIP

Roter and Hall (1992), in their book *Doctors talking with patients, patients talking with doctors*, describe four models of the doctor–patient relationship: paternalism, consumerism, default and mutuality.

The *paternalistic model* is characterized by high doctor/low patient control. The doctor makes decisions which he considers to be in the best interest of the patient; the patient cooperates with the advice and does as he is told. At certain times, this style of relationship is welcomed by the patient, for instance when the patient is seriously ill, vulnerable and unable to take part in a more equal relationship. It is also the preference of certain patients, especially among the elderly and less educated (Haug and Lavin 1983). However, there are questions about the appropriateness of this type of relationship, even when both patient and physician appear to agree with it. Patients and doctors are often on an unequal footing and few patients really have an effective role in shaping the relationship. A passive role may be the natural consequence of many years of deference without a full understanding of the alternatives (Deber 1994). It has been suggested that part of the doctor's role should be education and encouragement of patients to take part in adult–adult relationships with their physicians.

Consumerism is the other extreme. Here, there is low doctor/high patient control. A younger, better educated patient may take a more assertive role; the doctor may simply cooperate by acceding to the patient's requests for, say, investigation or medication. There are problems here too. Say that the patient's requests are outside normal practice, that they are not in the patient's best interests or are a waste of precious health care resources. In a health care system in which the patient as the consumer can exert his choice to change his doctor until he finds one who will accommodate his requests, and in which the doctor's income is dependent on attracting more patients and performing more tasks, good medical practice can be sacrificed on the altar of consumerism and financial incentive. In this model, trust between doctor and patient is eroded and the doctor's expertise is diminished just as the patient's is in the paternalistic model.

Default or laissez-faire describes a model in which no one takes responsibility, where both doctor and patient have low control and the relationship becomes aimless and unproductive for both parties.

In *mutuality*, there is both high doctor and high patient control. Patients' preferences are actively sought and compared explicitly to doctors' thoughts; doctors explain their reasoning in relation to patients' ideas. Open negotiation leads to a meeting of minds between two more equal parties and the production of a mutually agreed collaborative plan. A patient can openly explain which option he might prefer or why he might not choose or be able to follow a particular course of action. Similarly, the doctor can openly discuss her own dilemmas, explain why a patient's suggestion is not to the patient's advantage and why the doctor may not feel able to fulfil it. Often, both doctor and patient perspectives can be accommodated with minor adjustment; potential disagreements are discovered during the consultation and can be addressed then and there. In a more doctor-centred approach to planning, such doubts may not surface during the interview but appear later on, after the patient has left the room, to initiate the insidious process of non-adherence.

Mutuality can be promoted as a more reasonable starting position for the planning phase of the consultation than paternalism. At the very least, the patient should be invited to take an active part. As with information giving, a proportion of patients will not wish active involvement and will prefer physician dominance. The key is not to make assumptions but to openly discover patients' preferences for involvement in the process of shared decision making.

WHAT THEORETICAL EVIDENCE IS THERE TO SUPPORT THE COLLABORATIVE APPROACH TO PLANNING?

Many writers have provided theoretical support for the concept of a collaborative approach to planning. Herman (1985) stresses the importance of sharing possibilities and eliciting patient preferences so that patients understand their physician's rationale, are involved in decision making and share control with their physician. Quill (1983) discusses the role of negotiating and contracting in a consensual relationship. Slack (1977) argues that patients should be encouraged to make their own decisions with the aid of their physician rather than have the physician choose for them: doctors would then be freed from worrying about compliance (which implies 'following the doctor's orders') and from feeling responsible for all that occurs to their patients, from the liability that accompanies medical paternalism. Stewart *et al.* (1997) clearly support mutuality, collaboration and partnership in their model of patient-centred medicine.

Many authors now consider the term 'compliance' to be an outdated concept, with overtones of passivity and obedience. Instead, 'adherence' or more recently 'concordance' has been proposed, implying a more active collaborative role for the patient. It is proposed that this active involvement in decision making creates better patient understanding and commitment to plans, thereby reducing the likelihood of 'non-adherence' (Eisenthal *et al.* 1979; Meichenbaum and Turk 1987; Dye and DiMatteo 1995; Frank *et al.* 1995; Butler *et al.* 1996).

Coambs *et al.* (1995), in their recent review of the literature on non-compliance, conclude that of the models that have evolved to explain non-compliance, only those which incorporate patients' attitudes, health beliefs and intentions to comply – rather than patients' biological or social traits – have been successful in predicting non-compliance. They also conclude that 'when the patient–physician relationship is a negotiated process, in which there is increased understanding of and agreement upon a proposed treatment, higher levels of compliance with the therapeutic regime and improved health status can be achieved'.

Brody (1980) suggests four steps necessary to encourage mutuality. These suggestions bring together many of the ideas that are advocated throughout this book:

1 establishing an atmosphere conducive to participation, where contributions are welcomed and where the patient's ideas and questions are actively sought
2 ascertaining the patient's reasons for seeing the doctor and their goals and expectations
3 giving appropriate information about the nature of the problem, including the doctor's rationale, possible alternatives, their advantages and disadvantages and suggested recommendations (rather than directives)
4 eliciting the patient's informed suggestions and preferences and negotiating any disagreements.

Becker's (1974) health belief model shows how adherence to a regime of treatment or to a change in health behaviour is influenced by the balance between patients' understanding and appraisal of the potential benefits that might accrue and the costs and personal or social barriers to carrying out the proposed suggestions. In this model, the physician should not only educate the patient about the nature and effectiveness of treatments but also discover the patient's perceptions of costs and barriers so that these can be addressed and suggestions made to help overcome them. Only by a readiness to embrace a collaborative, negotiating approach to the consultation can this process be achieved.

Deber (1994) suggests that choosing the optimal treatment is often a marginal decision: the 'correct' decision is greatly influenced by the values that a particular patient attaches to different outcomes and to their perception of particular procedures. Only through knowledge of the patient's unique perspective of these issues can an informed and appropriate choice be made by patient and doctor together.

The research evidence to support the collaborative approach to planning

What research evidence do we have to demonstrate that a collaborative approach can improve patient outcomes?

Further to their work on the relationship between eliciting patient expectations and subsequent patient satisfaction, Eisenthal *et al.* (1979) demonstrated that higher levels of negotiation and patient participation in the decision-making process are associated with both increased adherence and satisfaction. By a negotiated approach, the authors meant eliciting patients' expectations and requests for care, actively negotiating treatment plans and checking negotiated plans to see if the patient agrees with them.

Schulman (1979) found that hypertensive patients who were more actively involved in treatment programmes had higher rates of adherence and more favourable treatment outcomes. Active involvement was defined as viewing themselves as collaborative partners, being involved in two-way communication and joint decision making, being informed of treatment rationales and being encouraged to voice opinions and report side-effects. 'Active' hypertensive patients demonstrated a better understanding of their illness, fewer side-effects, better adherence, greater adoption of health-promoting behaviour and, most importantly, better blood pressure control.

Brody *et al.* (1989) showed that patients reporting an active role in their medical visit were more satisfied with their doctors, had lower levels of illness concern and had a greater sense of control over their illness than passive patients.

Kaplan *et al.* (1989; 1996), in studies of chronic diseases (hypertension, insulin-dependent diabetes and rheumatoid arthritis) in both primary care and specialist settings, showed that patients whose physicians were less controlling and more participatory developed better functional status and better physiological outcomes. Patients of doctors who demonstrated a more participatory style were more satisfied and changed their doctors less frequently. They also demonstrated that patients who were more active in the consultation reported fewer health problems and functional limitations from their illness and rated their health more favourably. Active patients also achieved better control of their hypertension and diabetes. But were these findings due to intrinsic differences in patients' personalities? Or was patient activity itself the key to these physiological improvements and, if so, can such involvement in the consultation be improved by education?

To answer these questions Kaplan *et al.* therefore conducted a series of randomly controlled trials that separately looked at patients with hypertension, diabetes, breast cancer and ulcer disease. They investigated the effect of coaching patients in behavioural strategies to make them more active participants in the consultation. Patients were coached in how to improve their question asking, provided with techniques in negotiation and shown methods to decrease their embarrassment and fear of feeling foolish. They were also shown their own records and provided with algorithms to understand their treatment. These teaching interventions led to marked differences in the interview and its consequences. Patients were more active in the interview, made more contributions to the discussion, obtained more information from their physicians and, most importantly, achieved both better self-reported health and better physiological control of their illnesses (including lower diastolic blood pressure readings and lower HbA1 results). This improvement in physiological outcome has been replicated in diabetes by Rost *et al.* (1991). That these results have been obtained in a variety of chronic illnesses lends credence to this being a more generally applicable finding.

One interesting additional result was that more negative affect expressed by both physician and patient was related to better health outcomes. Negative affect in this context was defined as a broad spectrum of behaviours, including tension, anxiety, nervous laughter and self-consciousness as well as outright impatience or anger. This may well represent increased role tension induced by a change in the parties' normal relationship or, as Kaplan *et al.* have called it, 'healthy friction'. Or it may be that doctors who are more engaged with their patients appear more anxious or concerned. Whatever, patients afterwards expressed a significantly stronger preference for active involvement in medical decision making. Hall *et al.* (1981) also showed that increased physician negative affect is associated with increased patient satisfaction.

These findings confirm an earlier study by Roter (1977) which found that a simple ten-minute intervention prior to patients' consultations in primary care, in which patients were helped to ask questions of their physicians, led to a doubling of questions asked, a feeling of increased patient control and responsibility for their own health and less drop out from follow-up. Butow *et al.* (1994) showed that a question prompt sheet handed to patients ten minutes before an oncology appointment increased patient questioning about prognosis but not overall numbers of questions. Svarstad (1974) and Tuckett *et al.* (1985) have also shown that patients' willingness to ask questions or exhibit doubts leads to more information giving by doctors perhaps by alerting doctors to their patients' needs.

Fallowfield *et al.* (1990) found that women with breast cancer who were seen by surgeons who favoured offering patients a choice between mastectomy and lumpectomy suffered less anxiety and less depression than patients seen by surgeons who favoured either mastectomy or lumpectomy. This at first sight is strong support for the principle of allowing patients to share in decision making by allowing them choice. However, technical considerations prevented surgeons who favoured offering a choice from actually offering such a choice to 50% of their patients. Despite this, these patients still showed the same reduction in anxiety and depression as patients who were actually allowed to make a real choice. As Stewart (1995) comments: 'I would suggest that it was not just the decision-making power of the patient that was effective but rather the provision of a caring, respectful and empowering context in which a woman was enabled to make an important decision with both support and comfort.' This conclusion remains conjecture but certainly some aspect of the surgeon's ability to relate and communicate to the patient is apparently making a considerable difference to psychological outcome. Perhaps the willingness to share decision making is a reflection of these surgeons' shift towards a mutual rather than paternalistic model.

Stewart *et al.* (1997) have shown that interviews where patients perceived that the doctor and patient found common ground in the decision-making process (involving a mutual discussion of treatment options and goals and roles in management, checking for feedback, etc.) were associated with significantly fewer referrals and investigations over the two months following the interview. This suggests that a collaborative approach can reduce demands on the health care system.

It is a mistake to assume that all patients wish to be involved in a collaborative approach to planning; some feel more comfortable leaving decisions to their doctors (Cassileth *et al.* 1980; Strull *et al.* 1984; Blanchard *et al.* 1988; Ende *et al.* 1989; Sutherland *et al.* 1989; Beisecker and Beisecker 1990; Hack *et al.* 1994). For instance, in Strull *et al.*'s study of hypertensive out-patients, only 53% of patients wished to take an active part in decision making. In Blanchard *et al.*'s study of cancer patients, 92% wanted information but only 69% wanted to participate in decision making; 23% of those wanting full information still wished the doctor to make the decisions.

Deber *et al.* (1996) have recently questioned the results of previous studies that have shown low patient desire to participate in decision making. In their opinion, these studies failed to differentiate between the tasks of problem solving (requiring expertise and necessitating physician input) and decision making (where true choices involving trade-offs of advantages and disadvantages were available to the patient). In their own study, patients did not wish involvement in the former but mostly wished to be involved in the latter.

In Degner *et al.*'s (1997) study of 1012 women with a confirmed diagnosis of breast cancer attending hospital oncology clinics, 22% wanted to select their own cancer treatment, 44% wanted to select their treatment collaboratively with their doctors and 34% wanted to delegate this decision making to their doctors. Only 42% of women believed they had achieved their preferred level of control in decision making. The substantial difference between women's preferred and attained level of involvement in decision making suggests that we need to look more carefully at how we are dealing with this important aspect of communication and care.

The question that we need to address is how to discover each patient's individual wishes rather than make assumptions. Although older patients, less educated patients and those with more serious illnesses are more likely to prefer a non-participatory role, Strull *et al.* (1984) have demonstrated how difficult it is to guess each patient's desire for involvement in making decisions without enquiring directly. Rather than force all patients to adopt a collaborative role, it is the doctor's task to discover individual patients' preferences for participation and to tailor their approach accordingly. Since a patient's preferences for participation and information may vary depending on the nature or stage of the illness and the patient's personal development, preferences may need to be discussed periodically over time and from situation to situation.

Why should doctors share their ideas, thought processes and dilemmas?

One specific skill that contributes to a more collaborative and interactional approach to planning is sharing one's own thought processes, ideas and dilemmas. This offers advantages to doctor and patient alike:

- uncertainty is reduced and mutually understood common ground established. The patient begins to understand the rationale behind your suggestions and what the dilemmas are in a particular situation. The patient is not left guessing why you are proceeding along a certain path

- it encourages the patient to contribute their views. After your dilemmas are made apparent, the patient often contributes a statement that establishes their preference or gives further information helpful to your decision making. Sharing your ideas is a signal that you might be interested in hearing the patient's, thus encouraging more open communication
- it forces us to order our information giving. Often, we skip over diagnosis, aetiology and prognosis and go straight to treatment – the sharing approach helps prevent the omission of logical steps.

What skills can we recommend to learners to help them achieve a collaborative approach to planning?

Specific examples of these skills in action are:

- **Share own thoughts:** ideas, thought processes and dilemmas. *'There are two possibilities here which might explain your symptoms, either an ulcer or gallstones. It's not clear from just examining you which it is. I'm trying to decide between two ways forward – we can either just treat it as if it is an ulcer or we could do some tests first to get a more definite diagnosis.'*
- **Involve patient by making suggestions** rather than directives: *'My suggestion for tackling this would be ... What do you think?'*
- **Encourage patient to contribute their thoughts, ideas, suggestions:** *'I'd be interested to hear your thoughts about ways that I could help you to stop smoking.'*
- **Negotiate:** negotiates a mutually acceptable plan. *'What I've suggested makes sense to me ... but if it isn't right for you, we'll need to think again. Tell me what you feel about it.'*
- **Offer choices:** encourage patient where possible to make choices and decisions. *'There are several things we might try here, each as I've said with their own advantages and disadvantages ... Do you have any clear preference?'*
- **Check with patient:** if accepts plans, if concerns have been addressed. *'Now, can I just check that you are happy with the plan?'*

SECTION 5: OPTIONS IN EXPLANATION AND PLANNING

The four sections discussed above are common to all consultations featuring explanation and planning. We now discuss three optional elements which may or may not be applicable to any one interview:

1 if offering an opinion and discussing the significance of problems
2 if negotiating a mutual plan of action
3 if discussing investigations and procedures.

If offering an opinion and discussing the significance of problems

We have already discussed the evidence that doctors tend to discuss treatment and drug therapy while patients are more interested in diagnosis, prognosis and causation of their illness

(Helman 1981; Kindelan and Kent 1987) and that patients often come away from the medical interview without even basic information about their illness (Svarstad 1974; Boreham and Gibson 1978). Tuckett *et al.* (1985) have shown that patients' understanding and commitment to management plans are often poor because doctors seldom explain their rationale in any detail or provide explanations related to the patient's illness framework.

So what specific skills can we recommend to help you explain your opinion about a problem?

- Offer opinion of what is going on and name if possible
- Reveal rationale for opinion
- Explain causation, seriousness, expected outcome, short and long-term consequences
- Elicit patient's beliefs, reactions and concerns, e.g. if opinion matches patient's thoughts, acceptability, feelings.

A common example in practice demonstrates these skills in action:

'You've told me a lot about this pain in your elbow. I think the problem is tennis elbow ... and the reason why I think that this is the diagnosis is because ... Does that fit in with what you were thinking? All right, I think the reason why it might have come on now is because ... and it may give you discomfort for several months, I'm afraid. I don't think it's serious, and from what you've told me you are not concerned that it might be arthritis. How does that strike you?'

If negotiating a mutual plan of action

The specific skills that we can use for negotiating a plan of action are:

- discuss options, e.g. no action, investigation, medication or surgery, non-drug treatments (physiotherapy, walking aids, fluids, counselling), preventative measures
- provide information on action or treatment offered
  - name
  - steps involved, how it works
  - benefits and advantages
  - possible side-effects
- obtain patient's view of need for action, perceived benefits, barriers, motivation
- accept patient's views, advocate alternative viewpoint as necessary
- elicit patient's reactions and concerns about plans and treatments including acceptability
- take patient's lifestyle, beliefs, cultural background and abilities into consideration
- encourage patient to be involved in implementing plans, to take responsibility and be self-reliant
- ask about patient support systems, discuss other support available.

DISCUSSING AND OFFERING OPTIONS IN MANAGEMENT AND TREATMENT

Offering options is the first step in enabling patient choice. How can a patient with back pain choose whether to try physiotherapy, osteopathy, pain relief or rest without having the possible options clearly explained first?

PROVIDING INFORMATION ON ACTION OR TREATMENT OFFERED

Providing information about a proposed management or treatment is a highly skilled task. Take, for example, the scenario of prescribing hormone replacement therapy to a menopausal woman. Not only does the doctor have to give a clear explanation of how the treatment works and tailor his explanation to the patient's understanding and needs, he must also describe the risks and benefits of the treatment accurately, taking into account the patient's concerns. For instance, most women are concerned about the risk of breast cancer with hormone replacement therapy (Griffiths 1995), but are less knowledgeable about the benefits in terms of cardiovascular disease and stroke (Hope and Rees 1995). The doctor must describe and discuss the possible side-effects of the treatment, explain the different preparations available and explain how to take the preparation that the patient chooses.

OBTAINING THE PATIENT'S VIEW OF NEED FOR ACTION, PERCEIVED BENEFITS, BARRIERS AND MOTIVATION

Prevention and health promotion have become an important part of the doctor's domain (WHO 1985). Health workers in the fields of drug and alcohol addiction, smoking cessation and weight loss employ a number of useful psychological and communication models that enable them to maximize change in their clients' health-related behaviour. Priest and Speller (1991) cite three sets of skills in which a practitioner needs to be effective to help a patient change to a healthier lifestyle:

1 knowledge about risk factors
2 awareness and understanding about the patient's attitude to the problem affecting their health
3 knowledge and application of the skills involved in helping people to change.

Motivational interviewing. Motivational interviewing utilizes these three sets of skills to foster the individual's desire to change. In motivational interviewing, the practitioner's immediate task is to discover the patient's health beliefs as well as his readiness for change. Only then can the practitioner determine how best to work with each patient.

Motivational interviewing is based on the 'stages of change' model (Fig 5.1), originally designed by Prochaska and DiClemente (1986), and further developed in practice by Miller (1983) and van Bilson and van Emst (1989). The model describes a natural series of stages that people work through when considering change. It recognizes that at each of these stages people have different frames of mind and that professional intervention is more likely to be successful if tailored closely to whichever stage the individual is in at present. The practitioner's role is to discover where the patient is in the process of self-motivation and encourage and support their efforts. Patients' levels of confidence (in their ability to make the change) and conviction (regarding how convinced they are that the change is important) will also influence their success (Keller and Kemp White 1997). Motivational interviewing attempts to empower the patient to take responsibility for their own decisions by increasing their self-esteem and self-efficacy, by respecting their views and concerns and by negotiating suitable targets.

Useful texts which deal with motivational interviewing and the locus of control include: Miller and Rollnick (1991), Dye and DiMatteo (1995), Tate (1997), and Butler *et al.* (1996).

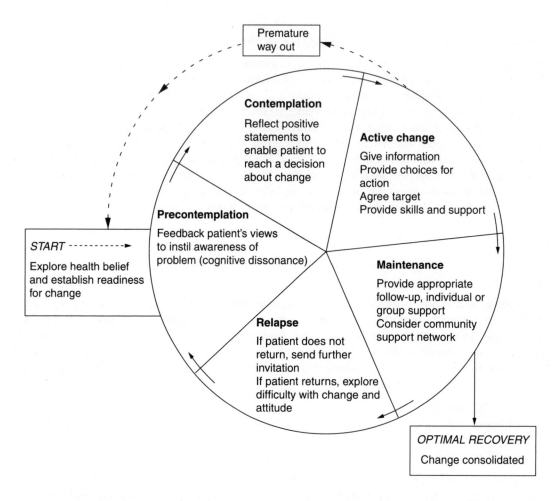

Fig 5.1 Intervention process using the 'stages of change' model (adapted from Prochaska and DiClemente 1986).

ACCEPTING PATIENT'S VIEWS: ADVOCATING AN ALTERNATIVE VIEWPOINT AS NECESSARY

A key skill that goes hand in hand with obtaining the patient's perspective is the accepting response, which we discussed in Chapter 4. This skill puts into action the key concept of initially accepting and acknowledging the legitimacy of patients' ideas without necessarily agreeing with them. Non-judgemental acceptance allows you later to offer your own perspective of the problem in the light of the patient's beliefs, discuss misperceptions, advocate a different approach if necessary and negotiate a mutually agreeable plan. But what if you feel that the patient's attitudes are seriously affecting their health yet they brush aside your suggestions? How can you challenge a firmly held belief without denigrating the patient?

Challenging and confronting patients (Box 5.2). Being honest in the medical interview can present difficulties for the doctor, particularly when faced with patients who appear not to be

---

Box 5.2 Confrontation

- Honestly bringing something of importance to someone's attention.
- Challenging a restricting attitude, belief or behaviour.
- Telling an uncomfortable truth.

Aim

- To allow the patient to hear you and acknowledge a problem while maintaining rather than destroying the relationship.
- To address the problem behaviour while affirming the patient's worth as a person.

Needs to be

- Honest
- True
- Supportive

The problem

Our own anxiety: our past experiences of confrontation (personal and professional) and the present situation lead us either to sledgehammer, pussyfoot or avoid.

Plan

- Signpost your intent.
- State what the problem is:
  - for you and the patient
  - what effect it is having.
- State what you would like to happen:
  - what benefits would then accrue to you both.
- Make a valuing statement about the person:
  - separate the person's behaviour from them as a person.
- Overtly demonstrate your care/empathy.
- Then give plenty of time, ask for the patient's feelings, move on into planning.

Adapted from Heron (1975)

---

confronting an important problem. Conflict with patients is usually unproductive and can leave the patient feeling both angry and unsupported. Contrast:

'You must stop smoking at once. You are a fool not to stop. I can't be responsible for what happens if you don't.'

with:

'I know that it is difficult for you to stop smoking at the moment ... you are going through a difficult period ... but your chest has got a lot worse in the last year and I'm concerned that you will continue to deteriorate this winter if you don't stop. What can we do to help you?'

Honesty and the ability to challenge beliefs in a constructive manner is an important part of enabling patients to change. Heron (1975), in his model of confronting and challenging a restrictive behaviour, suggests that the most effective approach is to give direct feedback within a caring context.

If discussing investigations and procedures

During the medical interview doctors often need to give information about investigations or procedures. Remember that what may seem trivial to the doctor may be highly alarming to the patient. A simple blood test may be terrifying. A two-week wait for the result of a mammogram for a patient who fears breast cancer can seem like a lifetime. Listening, empathy and achieving a shared understanding are all important. The key skills in this area of the consultation are:

- provide clear information on procedures including what patients may experience and how patients will be informed of results
- relate procedures to treatment plan: value and purpose
- encourage questions about and discussion of potential anxieties or negative outcomes.

Summary: explanation and planning is an interactive collaborative process

In much of this chapter we have advocated an interactive approach to explanation and planning: just giving information and dictating plans is clearly not enough. In Chapter 3, we discussed the limitations of direct transmission: if communication is viewed as a direct transmission process, the senders of messages assume that their responsibilities as communicators are fulfilled once they have formulated and sent a message. However, if communication is viewed as an interactive process, the interaction is complete only if the sender receives feedback about how the message is interpreted, whether it is understood and what impact it has on the receiver (Dance and Larson 1972).

We demonstrated that summarizing and checking are the key skills which enable this interactive approach to be put into practice in the information-gathering phase of the interview by providing feedback to the patient about what we think we have heard and understood. Now we have seen how further skills are required in the explanation and planning phase to ensure a similar degree of interaction.

Here we do not give a one-sided speech – to give information accurately, we need to check repeatedly whether we have made ourselves clear and whether the patient understands our thoughts before proceeding to the next chunk of information. We have seen how:

- a two-way interaction enables us to discover what information we have not yet provided
- asking the patient to restate the information they have just been told dramatically increases retention and understanding
- we need to give patients encouragement to ask questions, express doubts and seek clarification if we are to achieve a shared understanding, enhance patients' ability to make informed choices and prevent non-adherence

- we need to understand our patients' ideas if we want to align our explanations to patients' needs
- we need to involve the patient in planning by encouraging them to be part of the decision-making process and to voice their preferences.

We hope that this chapter has convinced you to continue the trend away from merely 'giving' information to patients and towards 'sharing' understanding and decision making. This shift promises not only more satisfying consultations for both patients and doctors but also better long-term health outcomes.

6

Closing the session

Introduction

Communication problems at the end of the consultation often relate to time issues. Just as you think that you have satisfactorily completed the interview and are drawing the session to an end, the patient introduces another major item. Just as you begin to organize follow-up arrangements, the patient asks a question that makes it clear that he has not understood any of your explanations so far. The doctor wants to close things down and push on to the next appointment; the patient seems keen to open things up again. These unmatched agendas easily lead to conflict and frustration.

What skills can we recommend to help with these problems? Difficulties in closure often emanate from communication issues occurring much earlier in the consultation. They can be avoided by attention to our use of communication skills during the beginning, information gathering and explanation and planning phases of the interview. Once these have been addressed, problems in this part of the consultation tend to evaporate.

But there are specific skills in the closing phase too. Summarizing and clarifying plans made and next steps for both parties, establishing what the patient should do if things do not go according to plan, checking that the patient is comfortable with follow-up arrangements, continuing to build the doctor–patient relationship – these are all essential elements of the consultation and contribute to improved understanding, adherence, satisfaction and health outcomes.

In this chapter we explore two separate but related questions:

1 What are the skills used throughout the rest of the consultation that can help closure to be more efficient?
2 What are the skills during closure itself that will help bring the consultation to a satisfactory end?

Objectives

Our objectives for this part of the interview may be summarized as:

- confirming the established plan of care
- clarifying next steps for both doctor and patient
- establishing contingency plans
- maximizing patient adherence and health outcomes
- making efficient use of time in the consultation
- continuing to encourage the patient to feel part of a collaborative process and to build the doctor–patient relationship for the future.

Again, these objectives encompass some of the tasks and check-points mentioned in other well-known guides to the consultation:

Byrne and Long (1976)	Phase 6: the consultation is terminated usually by the doctor.
Pendleton *et al.* (1984)	To use time and resources appropriately: (1) in the consultation (2) in the long term
Neighbour (1987)	Safety netting 'What if?' – consider what the doctor might do in each case
Cohen-Cole (1991)	Education, negotiation and motivation Developing rapport and responding to the patient's emotions
Keller and Carroll (1994)	Educating the patient Enlisting the patient in their own health care.

'What' to teach and learn about endings – the evidence for the skills

What actually happens in the closing segment of the interview?

White *et al.* (1994) have looked specifically at closure and have attempted to separate this element of the consultation from the explanation and planning phase. Listening to audiotapes of primary care physicians in Oregon, they identified closure by looking for sentences which demonstrated a transition from the educational to the ending phase; for example, 'OK, let's see you back in five months' or 'We'll just see how it goes in the future'. Their results were as follows:

- length of visits: av. 16.8 minutes
- length of closure: av. 1.6 minutes (1–9 minutes range)
- closure initiated by physician: in 86% of consultations
- new problems discussed not mentioned earlier in the visit: in 21% of closures
- physician behaviours in closure:
  - clarifying the plan (75%)
  - orientating the patient to next steps (56%)
  - providing information about the condition or therapy (53%)

– checking for understanding (34%)
– asking whether more questions (25%).

What behaviours earlier in the visit prevent new problems arising during closure?

White *et al.* (1994) found the following behaviours earlier in the visit tended to prevent new problems arising during closure:

- physicians using signposting to orientate patients to the flow of the visit ('Now I'm going to examine you and then we will have some time to discuss what's going on')
- physicians giving more information about the therapeutic regimen
- patients talking more about their therapy
- physicians asking for patients' beliefs and being more responsive to patients.

Barsky (1981) used the term 'hidden agendas' to describe problems that only surface in the closing moments of the interview. These are often emotionally charged or psychosocial issues and he surmised that such a late presentation of problems may well relate to the failure of the physician to facilitate disclosure earlier. Patients wait for the 'right' moment to present their 'real' problem; if it is not deliberately provided earlier on, the opportunity might not present itself until the very end of the interview.

In Chapter 2 we described Beckman and Frankel's (1984) key research on how our use of words and questions can easily and inadvertently direct the patient away from telling us their real reasons for coming to see us. Premature physician interruption and failure to screen for problems early on in the interview increase late-arising complaints.

What communication skills can we recommend in the earlier sections of the consultation that will aid efficient and satisfactory closure of the session?

Initiating the session

- Attentive listening
- Screening
- Agenda setting

Gathering information

- Signposting
- Exploring patients' ideas and concerns
- Addressing patients' feelings, thoughts and emotions
- Discussing psychosocial issues

Explanation and planning

- Information giving
- Involving patients in explanation and planning

- Checking for patients' understanding
- Asking for patients' questions.

What behaviours during closure are associated with inefficient endings?

White *et al.* (1994) discovered that the following behaviours during closure were associated with longer endings:

- physicians asking open questions
- physicians laughing, showing emotions, concern or responsiveness to patients
- patients engaging in psychological discussion, being friendly, dominant, responsive or in distress.

But are we trying to achieve a shorter closure? There is clearly a tension here between efficiency and completeness. If the doctor wishes to end the consultation more efficiently, one option would seem to be to behave in a more closed fashion. However, if the patient has further questions or hidden problems to discuss, closing them down will not maximize the full potential of the interview.

We should not abandon behaving in an open, collaborative and patient-centred way during closure. Our previous behaviour in the consultation will hopefully allow the patient at this stage to say 'No, I think you have answered all my questions' or 'No, I haven't any other problems'. But however well the consultation has proceeded, there will still be patients who leave their most embarrassing or worrying concern until the very end, until they have plucked up courage to broach it. We must not shut them out simply for the sake of short-term efficiency.

What are the specific elements of closure itself (Box 6.1)?

END SUMMARY

We looked at the value of internal summary during information gathering in Chapter 3. This essential tool is of great importance in this part of the consultation too. Summarizing the session briefly and clarifying the plan of care not only gives the physician and patient the chance to confirm their deliberations but can also act as a highly valuable facilitative tool,

---

Box 6.1 Skills for closing the interview

- **End summary:** summarizes session briefly and clarifies plan of care
- **Contracting:** contracts with patient re next steps for patient and physician
- **Safety netting:** safety nets appropriately – explains possible unexpected outcomes; what to do if plan is not working; when and how to seek help
- **Final checking:** checks that patient agrees and is comfortable with plan and asks if any corrections, questions or other items to discuss

allowing the patient to question or amend the physician's perceptions. Summarizing is an important aid to accuracy and hence to adherence. Remember always to leave space for the patient to make corrections or additions.

'So, just to recap, I think your diabetes has crept out of control a little over the last year, probably because of the weight that you have put on, but hopefully we'll be able to get your sugar back to a satisfactory level if you can get your weight down to where it was before. I'll find you the diet sheet that I mentioned and then we'll see you in two months and see how well you're managing. Is that a reasonable summary of what we've agreed?'

'Fine, doctor, although as I said I think it's the lack of exercise since my husband's heart attack that has been my downfall, and now he's a little better, perhaps I'll be able to get out walking more.'

CONTRACTING

Contracting with the patient about the next steps for both patient and physician allows each partner to identify their mutual roles and responsibilities (Stewart *et al.* 1997). The doctor may need to state explicitly how he will inform the patient of their results and what they should do in the meantime. The patient may need to confirm their willingness to adhere to the agreed treatment plan.

'So, I'll dictate a letter to the specialist explaining the problem and fax it later today. If there is anything unusual on the blood tests, I'll phone you before your appointment. Would you call me after your appointment and tell me what Dr Jones has said?'

SAFETY NETTING

Establishing contingency plans is a key step in closure. Explaining what the patient should do if things do not go according to plan, how they should contact you and what certain developments might mean provides important back-up. As Neighbour (1987) described, explaining possible unexpected outcomes and when and how to seek help are important steps not only in safe medical practice but also in relationship building. If you are told that your sore throat is tonsillitis and will get better with penicillin and it doesn't, you may well return later to another doctor in the practice who diagnoses glandular fever. You may then feel unhappy about the first partner's clinical acumen. However, if the first doctor had mentioned the possibility of glandular fever and that you should return for a blood test if the penicillin had not helped by the end of the course, your regard for the doctor may well have gone up as he correctly predicted the future.

FINAL CHECKING

As described above, it is important to check finally that the patient agrees and is comfortable with the plans that have been made and to ask if they have any corrections, questions or other items to discuss. Hopefully, the answer will be:

'No, that's just fine, thanks so much for helping me. You've answered all my questions.'

Summary

In this chapter, we have looked at the skills involved in closing the consultation. We have seen how the effectiveness of closure is related both to the appropriate use of communication skills in earlier sections of the consultation and also to the use of specific skills identified in this section of the *Calgary–Cambridge observation guide*. Summarizing, contracting, safety-netting and final checking all help to round off the interview safely, to establish mutually understood common ground, to reduce uncertainty for doctor and patient about both what has happened and what is expected in the future, and to complete the process of sharing, collaboration and partnership which we have promoted throughout this book.

The skills of closure enable patients to feel comfortable with a mutually agreed plan, to be clear about what will happen next and to move on with more confidence. The same skills enable doctors to complete the consultation more effectively and to start the next interview with less unfinished business or anxiety to undermine their concentration. We have already mentioned that the beginning of the consultation is often the root cause of many of the problems of closure. Here we see that without care and attention, closure can be the root cause of difficulties at the beginning of the next consultation. Putting aside the last patient is an important prerequisite for focusing attention on the next.

7

Relating specific issues to core communication skills

Introduction

In this final chapter, we look at specific communication issues in the medical interview. There are many issues and challenges for doctors when they communicate with patients. They range from death and dying to relating to patients of different ages and cultures, dealing with anger and aggression and difficulties with communication over the telephone. Here, we discuss briefly a selection of important issues and, in particular, explore the relationship between skills which are specific to a given issue and the core skills contained in the *Calgary–Cambridge observation guide* which have been the focus of the rest of this book.

The balance between issue-specific and core skills

Many of the recent books on communication in medicine devote the majority of their content to specific communication issues and give correspondingly less attention to core communication skills. In this book, we have reversed the balance. Learning and teaching about issues and core skills are both important. Why then have we concentrated primarily on core skills which doctors can use in all consultations? Our rationale is simple: most of the skills needed to deal with specific communication issues and challenges are contained in the set of core skills that we have already presented in Chapters 2–6. These core skills are the primary resource for dealing with all communication challenges; often all we need do to manage difficult communication issues is to apply these core skills carefully. If core skills are mastered first, more complex issues become very much easier to tackle.

Relating issue-specific skills to core skills

Many texts and teaching programmes do not underline the relationship between the skills needed in a specific situation and the relevant core skills (for example, relating the skills required in breaking bad news to the core skills of explanation and planning). Nor do they attempt to pull those skills into any sort of structure or framework which the learner can then use and remember for later occasions. In this chapter we offer an approach which relates issue-specific skills to core skills. To illustrate how important it is to have a thorough knowledge of the structure of the consultation and of appropriate core communication skills before adding in the specific skills related to a particular issue, we have chosen four issues which we think will be useful to all doctors. We explain the first issue, *breaking bad news*, in some depth. Three further examples – *cultural issues, interviewing psychotic patients* and *uncovering hidden depression* – are then discussed more briefly. At the end of this chapter we list a number of other communication issues and challenges for teachers and learners to tackle and useful sources where these issues are discussed in more depth. In our companion book on teaching and learning communication skills, we discuss how to incorporate the teaching and learning of specific issues into a skills-based curriculum.

Specific issues

Breaking bad news

The communication skills needed for breaking bad news are special variations on the core skills used in explanation and planning. The structure and skills of explanation and planning that we described in Chapter 5 provide a secure platform on which the issue-specific skills of breaking bad news can be superimposed. In fact, an understanding of the core skills alone provides almost all of the skills necessary to carry out this most important task. This is not surprising. The approach to explanation and planning that we have espoused in this book involves tailoring information giving to the patient's needs, attempting to understand the patient's perspective and working in a collaborative partnership, all skills that are important to breaking bad news. Tuckett *et al.*'s (1985) work demonstrates that information-giving skills are most required when there is a divergence between the doctor's and the patient's perspective; breaking bad news is the ultimate example of such a situation. Here the patient's hopes on entering the room are focused on the possibility, however faint, of receiving good news and the doctor has to gradually move the patient's attention towards the worrying facts that he must now begin to communicate.

This is one communication issue that most doctors appreciate to be a problem and find difficult. The psychological sequelae of breaking bad news in an abrupt and insensitive way can be devastating and long lasting (Finlay and Dallimore 1991) and over the years there have been numerous articles in the lay and medical press which illustrate doctors' deficiencies in this area. Hearteningly, Field (1995) has found that between '1983 and 1994, the amount and variety of teaching about death and dying in UK medical schools has grown considerably'. The same is true in Australia, North America and other parts of Europe. An increasing number of articles on how to teach breaking bad news have appeared in mainstream medical education journals over the same time period.

In both hospital and family practice, doctors may well have to tell patients that they have a serious or terminal condition; for example, that a patient has cancer or a positive HIV test or that a mother has a high risk of carrying a baby with Down's syndrome. More frequently, doctors have to tell the patient news which may not be considered to be particularly important or 'bad' to the practitioner but is perceived to be so to the patient. Examples include giving the diagnosis of rheumatoid arthritis or hypothyroidism, telling the patient that they are anaemic, giving the result of a mildly abnormal cervical smear or even telling a patient who wishes to go on holiday the next day that they have an influenza-like illness and are unlikely to be well in time to travel. So often as doctors we are unaware of the importance and likely effect on the patient of our information giving.

A FRAMEWORK FOR BREAKING BAD NEWS

Box 7.1 contains a framework for breaking bad news which is based on various people's work (Brod *et al.* 1986; Maguire and Faulkner 1988; Sanson-Fisher 1992; Buckman 1994; Cushing and Jones 1995).

THE RELATIONSHIP BETWEEN CORE AND ISSUE-SPECIFIC SKILLS IN BREAKING BAD NEWS

How does this framework for breaking bad news relate to the *Calgary–Cambridge observation guide* and the basic approach that we have proposed for the medical interview? The structure and skills described here mirror closely those that we outlined in Chapter 5 for explanation and planning and dovetail well with the objectives that we seek to achieve with any patient in this part of the consultation (see p. 92).

Key core skills
The key core skills for breaking bad news are common to all medical interviews:

- preparation
- summarizing
- negotiating an agenda
- listening
- picking up cues
- the use of silence
- discovering the patient's concerns and ideas
- encouraging the expression of feelings
- picking up the non-verbal cues
- building rapport
- empathy
- acceptance
- discovering the patient's starting point
- discovering the patient's feelings
- gauging what and how much information to give
- discovering whether a patient is a seeker or an avoider of information
- giving support
- giving clear jargon-free explanations
- chunking and checking information giving

(continued on p. 140)

Box 7.1   Suggestions for breaking bad news

Preparation

- Set up appointment as soon as possible.
- Allow enough uninterrupted time; if seen in surgery, ensure no interruptions.
- Use a comfortable, familiar environment.
- Invite spouse, relative, friend, as appropriate
- Be adequately prepared re clinical situation, records, patient's background.
- Doctor to put aside own 'baggage' and personal feelings wherever possible.

Beginning the session/setting the scene

- Summarize where things have reached to date; check with the patient.
- Discover what has happened since last seen.
- Calibrate how the patient is thinking/feeling.
- Negotiate an agenda.

Sharing the information

- Assess the patient's understanding first: what the patient already knows, is thinking or has been told.
- Gauge how much the patient wishes to know*.
- Give warning first that difficult information is coming, e.g. 'I'm afraid we have some work to do . . .'; 'I'm afraid it looks more serious than we had hoped …'
- Give basic information, simply and honestly; repeat important points.
- Relate your explanation to the patient's framework.
- Do not give too much information too early; do not pussyfoot but do not overwhelm.
- Give information in small 'chunks'; categorize information.
- Watch the pace; check repeatedly for understanding and feelings as you proceed.
- Use language carefully with regard given to the patient's intelligence, reactions, emotions; avoid jargon.

Being sensitive to the patient

- Read the non-verbal clues: face/body language, silences, tears.
- Allow for 'shut down' (when patient turns off and stops listening) and then give time and space; allow possible denial.
- Keep pausing to give the patient the opportunity to ask questions.
- Gauge the patient's need for further information as you go and give more information as requested, i.e. listen to the patient's wishes as patients vary greatly and one individual's preferences may vary over time or from one situation to another.
- Encourage expression of feelings and give early permission for them to be expressed, i.e. 'How does that news leave you feeling?'; I'm sorry that was difficult for you'; 'You seem upset by that'.

Box 7.1   Continued

- Respond to the patient's feelings and predicament with acceptance, empathy and concern.
- Check the patient's previous knowledge about information given.
- Specifically elicit all the patient's concerns.
- Check understanding of information given, e.g. 'Would you like to run through what you are going to tell your wife?'.
- Be aware of unshared meanings, e.g. what cancer means for the patient compared with what it means for the physician.
- Do not be afraid to show emotion or distress.

Planning and support

- Having identified all the patient's specific concerns, offer specific help by breaking down overwhelming feelings into manageable concerns, prioritizing and distinguishing the fixable from the unfixable.
- Identify a plan for what is to happen next.
- Give a broad timeframe for what may lie ahead.
- Give hope tempered with realism ('preparing for the worst and hoping for the best').
- Ally yourself with the patient ('We can work on this together … between us'), i.e. co-partnership with the patient/advocate of the patient.
- Emphasize the quality of life.
- Safety net.

Follow-up and closing

- Summarize and check with the patient.
- Do not rush the patient to treatment.
- Set up early further appointment, offer telephone calls, etc.
- Identify support systems; involve relatives and friends.
- Offer to see/tell spouse or others.
- Make written materials available.

Remember doctor's anxiety re giving information, previous experience, failure to cure or help

---

* Various authors make different recommendations about how this task should be accomplished. Buckman (1994) suggests a direct preliminary question such as 'If this condition turns out to be something serious, are you the type of person who likes to know exactly what is going on?'. Maguire and Faulkner (1988) suggest a hierarchy of euphemisms for the bad news, pausing after each to gain the patient's reaction. Other authors suggest making a more direct start to giving the news after a warning shot and gauging how to proceed as you go; they argue that patients who wish to use denial mechanisms will still be able to blank out what they do not want to hear.

- relating explanations to the patient's framework
- checking understanding
- giving opportunity to ask questions
- planning
- offering support
- safety netting.

Giving a warning shot first. This is a special case of signposting information that is about to be given. It alerts the patient. There are a number of ways to do this; which might be the best in the circumstance depends on the patient's situation and the doctor's style. For the patient with a terminal illness or a threatened miscarriage awaiting the result of a scan, it might be *'I'm afraid the news isn't as good as we hoped'* accompanied by appropriate body language. The doctor can then pause and let the likelihood of the news being difficult for the patient sink in before continuing the interview.

Key issue-specific skills
The main issue-specific skills for breaking bad news can be thought of as 'add on' skills, to be superimposed on the core skills described above.

How to set up the appointment. If the news is serious and complex information needs to be given, this requires special thought and planning. When and where should it be done? Who should be there? Are you as the doctor thoroughly prepared emotionally and factually?

When to stop for the 'shutdown'. Acknowledging that the patient does not wish to hear any more requires chunking and checking of your information giving as you proceed and picking up verbal cues (for example, changing the subject abruptly) or, more commonly, non-verbal cues (the patient becoming silent or looking uncomfortable or angry).

Interviewing more than one person at a time. Many ill people or people who know that they are going to be given difficult or complicated information bring a relative or friend with them to see the doctor. You then have more than one patient present with different ideas, concerns and expectations and different agendas. Focusing on the 'main' patient is essential. When there is time it is often helpful to agree to see the patient and relatives both separately and together. Note the results of Benson and Britten's (1996) study of patients with cancer which showed that most rejected disclosure to others without their consent.

Co-partnership and advocacy. Support for the patient is essential. Overt statements such as *'We need to work on this together'* or *'I will undertake to speak to the specialist on your behalf ...'* or *'You will not be left to cope with this on your own ... How can we go forward now?'* are examples of phrasing which may help patients.

Giving hope tempered with realism. This is easier for the doctor when the patient has a real hope of recovery or improvement, for example a patient recovering from a road traffic accident or a patient who is found to have a renal calculus. It is much more difficult to give hope to a patient who has suffered a severe stroke or for whom chemotherapy has failed. It is important for the doctor to discover the patient's own coping strategies here and to find out how optimistic a person they usually are. Doctors are not gods and they are often mistaken in the prognoses they give. All patients need hope and the key to giving it is to base it realistically on the patient's situation and their feelings about it.

Doctors not hiding their own distress. Patients can be upset by doctors who remain unmoved by their distress at being given bad news (Woolley *et al.* 1989). Doctors should not fear displaying emotion (Fallowfield 1993). But how much of your own distress to share with a patient is a difficult judgement to make and must depend on individual personalities and situations at the time. Clearly, it is not the patient's task to care for the doctor's distress. Building the relationship with the patient is the overall objective here.

Note that even the issue-specific skills described above fit into the five-task structure of our guide. How to set up the appointment belongs under initiation and gathering information, giving a warning shot and when to stop for shut down under explanation and planning, and the rest under building the relationship.

We suggest that doctors keep the tasks of explanation and planning in mind as they proceed through the interview and continually ask themselves the following:

- Am I in a position to give this patient accurate information?
- Have I discovered the patient's illness framework and, in particular, his thoughts and feelings and what he already knows?
- Have I developed sufficient rapport with the patient?
- What is the effect on the patient of what I am saying?
- Am I going at the patient's pace?
- Am I being flexible and supportive?
- Am I negotiating an effective plan for the future?

Cultural issues

The communication skills needed for exploring multicultural issues are a special case of the core skills used in understanding the patient's perspective (in gathering information and in explanation and planning) and in relationship building.

Many of the concepts which helped formulate the disease–illness model (as discussed in Chapter 3) came originally from anthropological and cross-cultural studies. Multicultural interviews were viewed as an extreme example of all medical encounters and the lessons learned were later applied to doctors and patients from the same culture. Here we are reversing the process and exploring how the core skills of discovering the patient's illness framework apply to the specific difficulties of the multicultural situation where doctors and patients often hold differing cultural perspectives.

Increasingly, we encounter ethnic complexities and mobility of peoples throughout the world. Johnson and colleagues (1995) have said that 'each culture is a textured pattern of beliefs and practices, some of which are coherent and consistent and others contested and contradictory'. They suggest that doctors must explore a patient's health beliefs and views of their symptoms and illness in every medical interview. If doctors ignore this advice, they risk making assumptions or value judgements and stereotyping patients. This can lead not only to conflict but also inaccuracy.

Johnson and colleagues also make the following points which doctors may find useful when consulting with a patient who comes from a culture different from their own: a patient's culture provides her with ideas about health and illness, notions about causality, beliefs about who controls health-care decisions and how steps in seeking health care are made. Johnson *et al.* have also developed a useful explanatory model which sets out common differences between Western-trained physicians and traditional ethnic patients. This approach is supported by a cross-cultural study by Chugh *et al.* (1993). Their main findings were that there were a number of barriers to patient satisfaction, to doctors giving diagnosis and treatment and to patients receiving it. The barriers were related to the patient's cultural experiences, ideas, beliefs and expectations as well as language difficulties.

Myerscough (1992) and Eleftheriadou (1996) give some excellent and detailed information about a number of problems related to culture that are commonly encountered by Western physicians. Examples given include the importance of the family structure and lifestyle, women's roles, attitudes towards women and their children, dress, religion, food and fasting, and life and death.

Some knowledge of the different ethnic cultures in which a physician practises is useful and in some cases it is vital. But the core skills of understanding each individual patient and their particular health beliefs, whichever culture they come from, remain essential. Some knowledge and familiarity undoubtedly gives the doctor confidence and may allow some 'short cuts' to be made. But labelling the patient with the attitudes and outlook of a whole race or culture may be just as damaging as not being sensitive to multicultural issues at all; the doctor's objective must be to find out each individual patient's unique perspective and experience of illness (Chugh *et al.* 1994). This is just as important when both doctor and patient apparently share the same culture.

KEY CORE SKILLS

Although these skills relate mainly to understanding the patient's perspective during both information gathering and explanation and planning, skills of relationship building also pertain to:

- checking pronunciation of name and how the patient would like to be addressed
- discovering the patient's ideas, concerns, expectations of medical diagnosis and treatment
- non-judgemental acceptance of ideas and beliefs
- sensitivity to feelings and emotions
- demonstrating interest, concern and respect
- empathy
- sensitivity during the physical examination
- picking up verbal and non-verbal cues
- clarity in giving information
- checking understanding
- relating explanations to patient's illness framework
- negotiating an approach to management
- checking if concerns have been addressed.

KEY ISSUE-SPECIFIC SKILLS

- willingness to explore and understand cultural differences (related to social, religious, and health practices and beliefs)
- sensitivity to the patient's wish to be interviewed with a family member
- interviewing more than one patient at a time

- willingness to understand different family and marital relationships
- awareness of the possibility of cultural differences in non-verbal communication patterns
- offering choices, for example the examination of a female patient by a doctor of the same gender
- offering the help of an interpreter and handling an interpreter in the interview
- understanding social and community networks.

Some examples of possible phrasing include:

'I'm not familiar with the culture which you come from … Please tell me if there are things that are important to you when you go into hospital so I can tell the doctors who will be looking after you. I want to make things easier for you …'
'I can understand that it must be frustrating for you that I can't understand you as well as you would like. Would it help if we had an interpreter?'
'I'd like to know what sort of treatment you were expecting … or hoping for. From what I know of your culture, it might be quite different from what we offer here, and I'd like to help.'

Eleftheriadou (1996) provides a concise and practical summary of what to consider when communicating with patients from different cultures and offers some particularly useful examples of how to improve that communication.

Mental illness: psychosis and hidden depression

Interviewing patients with mental illness demonstrates the importance of the core skills of gathering information (in particular, of taking an accurate clinical history) and building the relationship.

THE PSYCHOTIC PATIENT

Psychotic patients present particular challenges. Here the patient is out of touch with reality; this may be quite a subtle state or the patient may be acutely ill and out of control. Not only may such patients be unable to function normally but their communication skills are impaired and they are commonly frightened and untrusting. Their anxious and sometimes angry relatives and friends may complicate the interviewing process. The beginning of an interview with a psychotic patient is crucial; lack of mutual trust and rapport in the first minute or two can quickly lead to conflict and difficulties. Gathering information in a sensitive and empathic manner when the doctor himself is frightened requires communication skills of a high order. Davies (1997) has suggested that the use of open questions initially is vital in elucidating the nature of the presenting problem and establishing rapport. Asking directive or closed questions is not easy, yet as Cox *et al.* (1989) have demonstrated, more information may be elicited if the interviewer makes specific probes in their directive questioning and uses the open-to-closed cone effectively (see Chapter 3 on gathering information).

The *key core skills* needed to achieve these aims include:

- listening
- using the open-to-closed cone
- picking up cues
- gauging the patient's emotional state

- asking directive questions
- clarifying
- signposting
- eliciting the patient's ideas and concerns and the effects of the illness on his life
- proceeding at the patient's pace
- all the skills needed to build the relationship.

When clarifying what the patient is saying and the current context of the patient's illness, taking a non-critical approach can be helpful:

'I'm finding it difficult to understand what you are saying at the moment. Could I ask some questions which will help to make things clearer?'

Two important communication challenges with psychotic patients are accurate assessment of the mental state and negotiating treatment. The *key issue-specific skills* include those that assess the patient's mood (accurate observation of the patient's non-verbal behaviour; asking sensitively how the patient is feeling), those that assess the patient's disordered beliefs and thinking processes and those that assess the patient's insight into his illness. Gathering information from others and interviewing a friend or relative together with a psychotic patient is not easy. The doctor needs to be calm and steady in her approach. Being the advocate of the patient at the same time as challenging and confronting him with his illness is a real skill.

When assessing the patient's disordered beliefs and thinking processes, the following phrases may come in useful:

'I'm wondering what you were thinking when you said ...'
'You said that people were controlling you through the television. Can you tell me a bit more about that?'
or the more direct
'Do you have thoughts that you hear out loud in your head?'
or
'Do you feel you have special powers?'

When assessing the patient's insight into his illness, use signposting and sensitive phrasing of specific direct questions, for example:

'You've told me that you are hearing voices again. I remember last time you were ill, and the same thing was happening ... what do you think?'

Combining advocacy and support with challenge is a difficult balancing act with a psychotic patient. It is helpful for the doctor to find phrases that work well in different circumstances and to practise them:

'I know that you feel that you are not ill at the moment, but I am concerned about you today ... I think that you need some treatment and I would like to help.'

When gathering information from others it is often very important to get accurate information from those who know the patient well. This can be perceived as threatening and unsupportive to a paranoid person with disordered thinking and it is important to have the patient's permission if the doctor is aiming to achieve a collaborative relationship.

Uncovering hidden depression and assessing suicidal risk

Depression is a frequently occurring psychiatric disorder which is easily missed in medical practice. Accurate diagnosis depends on the skill of the doctor. Again, uncovering and assessing depression in patients is a special case of gathering information and building the relationship.

KEY CORE AND ISSUE-SPECIFIC SKILLS

The key core and issue-specific skills required for interviewing depressed and suicidal patients are very similar to those for psychotic patients. As well as using the core skills from Chapters 3 and 4 which encourage the patient to 'open up', it is essential to discover whether the depressed patient has a severe and sustained disturbance of mood accompanied by feelings of worthlessness, loss of interest, and morbid guilt together with alterations in appetite, weight and sleep pattern. Patients who are thought to be a suicidal risk must be asked specifically about thoughts of hopelessness, self-harm, death or suicide. It is often possible to ask a direct question, or it may be appropriate to ask it in a more oblique fashion, 'testing the water' first. For example:

'I'm wondering how low you really are. Can you bear to tell me?'
'You look depressed today. Would you like to tell me about how you are feeling?'
'You are wondering if you are depressed. I'd like to ask you some specific questions about your mood, concentration, appetite and sleeping patterns which will help us find out.'
'Do you ever feel that there's a light at the end of the tunnel?'
'You've told me how difficult it is to sleep. What is going through your mind when you are lying tossing and turning?'
'Some people feel that they can't go on when they are depressed. Have you had thoughts like that, that you'd like to end it all?'

Other specific issues, contexts and challenges

Many other communication issues in medicine can be usefully explored in a similar way, again relating the core skills (which are described in the *Calgary–Cambridge observation guide* and elaborated upon in Chapters 2–6) to the particular issue-specific skills required for the particular issue or challenge:

- ethical issues
- gender issues
- age-related issues – interviewing children, adolescents or the elderly
- prevention and health promotion issues
- talking with patients whose communication is impaired
- low literacy patients
- uncommunicative patients
- talking to relatives and other third parties
- telephone interviews

- communication during ward rounds
- death, dying and bereavement
- somatization
- anger and aggression
- handling complaints
- malpractice
- identifying emotional and psychosocial problems
- taking a sexual history
- interviewing a person with AIDS
- interviewing and intervention for alcohol and other addictive problems
- talking with patients in intensive medicine – acute life-threatening disease or injury
- ending the unsatisfactory doctor–patient relationship.

Further reading

Breaking bad news

Good discussions and teaching examples of breaking bad news in the literature include:

Buckman R (1994) *How to break bad news: a guide for health care professionals*. Papermac, London.

Buckman R (1996) Talking to patients about cancer. *BMJ*. **313**: 699–701.

Cushing AM and Jones A (1995) Evaluation of a breaking bad news course for medical students. *Med Educ*. **29**: 430–5.

Fallowfield L (1993) Giving sad and bad news. *Lancet*. **341**: 476–8.

Fallowfield LJ and Lipkin M (1995) Delivering sad or bad news. In *The medical interview: clinical care, education and research* (eds M Lipkin *et al.*). Springer-Verlag, New York.

Faulkner A, Argent J, Jones A *et al.* (1995) Improving the skills of doctors in giving distressing information. *Med Educ*. **29**: 303–7.

Lloyd M and Bor R (1996) *Communication skills for medicine*. Churchill Livingstone, Edinburgh.

Maguire P (1991) Managing difficult communication tasks. In *Developing communication and counselling skills in medicine* (ed R Corney). Tavistock/Routledge, London and New York.

Maguire P and Faulkner A (1988) Communicate with cancer patients. 1. Handling bad news and difficult questions. 2. Handling uncertainty, collusion and denial. *BMJ*. **297**: 907–9 and 972–4.

Poingdestre D (1995) Terminal illness. In *Counselling in primary health care* (eds J Keithley and G Marsh). Oxford University Press, Oxford.

Ptacek JT and Eberhardt TL (1996) Breaking bad news: a review of the literature. *JAMA*. **276**(6): 496–502.

Cultural issues

Eleftheriadou Z (1994) *Transcultural counselling*. Central Book Publishing, London.

Helman CG (1994) *Culture, health and illness*. Butterworth-Heinemann, Oxford.

Johnson TM, Hardt EJ and Kleinman A (1995) Cultural factors. In *The medical interview: clinical care, education and research* (eds M Lipkin *et al.*). Springer-Verlag, New York.

Kleinman A, Eisenberg L and Good B (1978) Culture, illness and care: clinical lessons from anthropological and cross-cultural research. *Ann Intern Med.* **88**: 251–8.

Myerscough PR (1992) *Talking with patients*. Oxford University Press, Oxford.

Mental illness: psychosis and hidden depression

Blacker R (1991) The diagnosis of patients at risk of psychiatric disorder. In *Developing communication and counselling skills in medicine* (ed R Corney). Routledge, London and New York.

Cohen-Cole SA (1991) *The medical interview: the three-function approach*. Mosby Year Book, St Louis.

Cohen-Cole SA and Mance R (1995) Interviewing the psychotic patient and interviewing the suicidal patient. In *The medical interview: clinical care, education and research* (eds M Lipkin *et al.*). Springer-Verlag, New York.

Forth C (1995) Psychiatric disorders. In *Counselling in primary health care* (eds J Keithley and G Marsh). Oxford University Press, Oxford.

Geisler L (1991) *Doctor and patient – a partnership through dialogue; new ways of mutual understanding* (translator JM Massey). Pharma Verlag, Frankfurt.

Other specific issues, contexts and challenges

Brewin T (1996) *Relating to the relatives: breaking bad news, communication and support*. Radcliffe Medical Press, Oxford.

Corney R (ed) (1991) *Developing communication and counselling skills in medicine*. Tavistock/Routledge, London.

Faulkner A and Maguire P (1994) *Talking to cancer patients and their relatives*. Oxford University Press, Oxford.

Fielding R (1995) *Clinical communication skills*. Hong Kong University Press.

Geisler L (1991) *Doctor and patient – a partnership through dialogue; new ways of mutual understanding*. (translator JM Massey). Pharma Verlag, Frankfurt.

Hope T, Fulford KM and Yates A (1996) *The Oxford practice skills course: ethics, law and communication skills in health care education*. Oxford University Press, Oxford.

Keithley J and Marsh G (1995) *Counselling in primary health care*. Oxford University Press, Oxford.

Kubler-Ross E (1967) *On death and dying*. Tavistock Publications, London.

Lipkin M, Putman SM and Lazare A (eds) (1995) *The medical interview: clinical care, education and research.* Springer-Verlag, New York.

Lloyd M and Bor R (1996) *Communication skills for medicine.* Churchill Livingstone, Edinburgh.

Myerscough PR (1992) *Talking with patients.* Oxford University Press, Oxford.

Parkes CM (1972) *Bereavement; studies of grief in adult life.* International Universities Press, Inc., New York.

Tate P (1997) *The doctor's communication handbook* (2nd edn). Radcliffe Medical Press, Oxford.

The Professional Education and Training Committee of New South Wales Cancer Council and the Post-graduate Medical Council of New South Wales (1992) *Communicating with your patients: an interactional skills training manual for junior medical officers.*

References

Arborelius E and Bremberg S (1992) What can doctors do to achieve a successful consultation? Video-taped interviews analysed by the 'consultation map' method. *Fam Prac*. **9**: 61–6.

Argyle M (1975) *Bodily communication*. International Universities Press, New York.

Baker SJ (1955) The theory of silences. *J Gen Psychol*. **53**: 145.

Barrows HS and Tamblyn RM (1981) *Problem based learning: an approach to medical education*. Springer Publishing House, New York.

Barsevich AM and Johnson JE (1990) Preference for information and involvement, information-seeking and emotional responses of women undergoing colposcopy. *Research in Nursing and Health*. **13**: 1–7.

Barsky AJ (1981) Hidden reasons some patients visit doctors. *Ann Intern Med*. **94**: 492-8.

Bass LW and Cohen RL (1982) Ostensible versus actual reasons for seeking pediatric attention: another look at the parental ticket of admission. *Pediatrics*. **70**: 870–4.

Becker MH (1974) The health belief model and sick role behaviour. *Health Education Monograph*. **2**: 409–19.

Beckman HB and Frankel RM (1984) The effect of physician behaviour on the collection of data. *Ann Intern Med*. **101**: 692–6.

Beckman HB, Frankel RM and Darnley J (1985) Soliciting the patients complete agenda: a relationship to the distribution of concerns. *Clin Res*. **33**: 714A.

Beisecker A and Beisecker T (1990) Patient information-seeking behaviours when communicating with doctors. *Med Care*. **28**: 19–28.

Benson J and Britten N (1996) Respecting the autonomy of cancer patients when talking with their families: qualitative analysis of semi-structured interviews with patients. *BMJ*. **313**: 729–31.

Berg JS, Dischler J, Wagner DJ *et al.* (1993) Medication compliance: a health care problem. *Ann Pharmacotherapy*. **27**: 3–22.

Bertakis KD (1977) The communication of information from physician to patient: a method for increasing patient retention and satisfaction. *J Fam Prac*. **5**: 217–22.

Bertakis KD, Roter D and Putnam SM (1991) The relationship of physician medical interview style to patient satisfaction. *J Fam Prac*. **32**: 175–81.

Blacker R (1991) The diagnosis of patients at risk of psychiatric disorder. In *Developing communication and counselling skills in medicine* (ed R Corney). Routledge, London and New York.

Blacklock SM (1977) The symptom of chest pain in family medicine. *J Fam Prac*. **4**: 429–33.

Blanchard CG, Labrecque MS, Ruckdeschel JC *et al.* (1988) Information and decision-making preferences of hospitalised adult cancer patients *Soc Sci Med*. **27**: 1139.

Boreham P and Gibson D (1978) The informative process in private medical consultations: a preliminary investigation. *Soc Sci Med*. **12**: 409–16.

Bourhis RY, Roth S and MacQueen G (1989) Communication in the medical setting: a survey of medical and everyday language use amongst patients, nurses and doctors. *Soc Sci Med*. **28**: 339–46.

Bradshaw PW, Ley P, Kincey JA *et al.* (1975) Recall of medical advice: comprehensibility and specificity. *Br J Soc Clin Psychol*. **14**: 55–62.

Briggs GW and Banahan BF (1979) *A training workshop in psychological medicine for teachers of family medicine*. Handouts 1–3: Therapeutic communication. Society of Teachers of Family Medicine, Denver, CO.

Brod TM, Cohen MM and Weinstock E (1986) *Cancer disclosure: communicating the diagnosis to patients – a video-tape*. Medcom, Inc., Garden Grove, CA.

Brody DS (1980) The patient's role in clinical decision-making. *Ann Intern Med*. **93**: 718–22.

Brody DS and Miller SM (1986) Illness concerns and recovery from a URI. *Med Care*. **24**: 742–8.

Brody DS, Miller SM, Lerman CE *et al.* (1989) Patient perception of involvement in medical care: relationship to illness attitudes and outcomes. *J Gen Intern Med*. **4**: 506–11.

Broyles S, Sharp C, Tyson J *et al.* (1992) How should parents be informed about major procedures? An exploratory trial in the neonatal period. *Early Hum Dev*. **31**: 67–75.

Buckman R (1994) *How to break bad news: a guide for health care professionals*. Papermac, London.

Buller MK and Buller DB (1987) Physicians' communication style and patient satisfaction. *J Health Soc Behav*. **28**: 375–88.

Burack RC and Carpenter RR (1983) The predictive value of the presenting complaint. *J Fam Prac*. **16**: 749–54.

Butler C, Rollnick S and Stott N (1996) The practitioner, the patient and resistance to change: recent ideas on compliance. *Can Med Assoc*. **154** (9): 1357–62.

Butow PN, Dunn SM, Tattersall MHN *et al.* (1994) Patient participation in the cancer consultation: evaluation of a question prompt sheet. *Ann Oncol*. **5**: 199–204.

Byrne PS and Long BEL (1976) *Doctors talking to patients*. Her Majesty's Stationery Office, London.

Campion PD, Butler NM and Cox AD (1992) Principal agendas of doctors and patients in general practice consultations. *Fam Prac*. **9**: 181–90.

Carroll JG and Monroe J (1979) Teaching medical interviewing: a critique of educational research and practice. *J Med Educ*. **54**: 498–500.

Cassata DM (1978) Health communication theory and research: an overview of the communication specialist interface. In *Communication yearbook* (ed BD Ruben). Transaction Books, New Brunswick, NJ.

Cassell EJ (1985) *Talking with patients*. Vol 2. *Clinical technique*. MIT Press, Cambridge, MA.

Cassileth B, Zupkis R and Sutton-Smith K (1980) Information and participation preferences among cancer patients. *N Engl J Med.* **162**: 169–76.

Chugh U, Dillman E, Kurtz SM *et al.* (1993) Multicultural issues in medical curriculum: implications for Canadian physicians. *Med Teacher.* **15**: 83–91.

Chugh U, Agger-Gupta N, Dillman E *et al.* (1994) *The case for culturally sensitive health care: a comparative study of health beliefs related to culture in six North-east Calgary communities.* Research report. Citizenship & Heritage Secretariat, Calgary, Alberta.

Coambs RB, Jensen P, Hoa Her M *et al.* (1995) Review of the scientific literature on the prevalence, consequences, and health costs of noncompliance and inappropriate use of prescription medication in Canada. Pharmaceutical Manufacturers Association of Canada (University of Toronto Press), Ottawa.

Cohen-Cole SA (1991) *The medical interview: the three-function approach.* Mosby Year Book, St Louis.

Corney R (ed) (1991) *Developing communication and counselling skills in medicine.* Tavistock/Routledge London.

Cox A (1989) Eliciting patients' feelings. In *Communicating with medical patients* (eds M Stewart and D Roter). Sage Publications, Inc., Newbury Park, CA.

Cox A, Hopkinson K and Rutter M (1981*a*) Psychiatric interviewing techniques. II. Naturalistic study. *Br J Psychiat.* **138**: 283–91.

Cox A, Rutter M and Holbrook D (1981*b*) Psychiatric interviewing techniques V. Experimental study. *Br J Psychiat.* **139**: 29–37.

Cushing AM and Jones A (1995) Evaluation of a breaking bad news course for medical students. *Med Educ.* **29**: 430–35.

Dance FEX (1967) Toward a theory of human communication. In *Human communication theory: original essays* (ed FEX Dance). Holt, Rinehart and Winston, New York.

Dance FEX and Larson CE (1972) *Speech communication: concepts and behavior.* Holt, Rinehart and Winston, New York.

Davies T (1997) ABC of mental health: mental health assessment. *BMJ.* **314**: 1536–9.

Deber R (1994) The patient–physician partnership: changing roles and the desire for information. *Can Med Assoc.* **151**: 171–6.

Deber R, Kraetschmer N and Irvine J (1996) What role do patients wish to play in treatment decision-making? *Arch Intern Med.* **156**: 1414–20.

Degner LF, Kristjanson LJ, Bowman D *et al.* (1997) Information needs and decisional preferences in women with breast cancer. *JAMA.* **277**: 1485–92.

DeVito JA (1988) *Human communication: the basic course* (4th edn). Harper & Row, New York.

Deyo RA and Diehl AK (1986) Patient satisfaction with medical care for low back pain. *Spine.* **11**: 28–30.

DiMatteo MR, Taranta A, Friedman HS *et al.* (1980) Predicting patient satisfaction from physicians' non-verbal communication skill. *Med Care.* **18**: 376–87.

DiMatteo MR, Hays RD and Prince LM (1986) Relationship of physicians' non-verbal communication skill to patient satisfaction, appointment non-compliance, and physician workload. *Health Psychol.* **5**: 581–94.

Dye NE and DiMatteo MR (1995) Enhancing cooperation with the medical regimen. In *The medical interview* (eds M Lipkin, SM Putnam and A Lazore). Springer-Verlag, New York.

Egan G (1990) *The skilled helper: a systematic approach to effective helping.* Brooks/Cole, Pacific Grove, CA.

Egbert LD, Batitt GE, Welch CE *et al.* (1964) Reduction of postoperative pain by encouragement and instruction of patients. *N Engl J Med.* **270**: 825–7.

Eisenthal S and Lazare A (1976) Evaluation of the initial interview in a walk-in clinic. *J Nervous and Mental Disease.* **162**: 169–76.

Eisenthal S, Emery R, Lazare A *et al.* (1979) 'Adherence' and the negotiated approach to parenthood. *Arch Gen Psychiat.* **36**: 393.

Eisenthal S, Koopman C and Stoeckle JD (1990) The nature of patients' requests for physicians' help. *Academic Med.* **65**: 401–5.

Ekman P, Friesen WV and Ellsworth P (1972) *Emotion in the human face: guidelines for research.* Pergamon, New York.

Eleftheriadou Z (1996) Communicating with patients of different backgrounds. In *Communication skills for medicine* (eds M Lloyd and R Bor). Churchill Livingstone, Edinburgh.

Ely JW, Levinson W, Elder NC *et al.* (1995) Perceived causes of family physicians' errors – see comments. *J Fam Prac.* **40**(4): 337–44.

Ende J, Kazis L, Ash AB *et al.* (1989) Measuring patients' desire for autonomy. *J Gen Intern Med.* **4**: 23–30.

Evans BJ, Stanley RO, Mestrovic R *et al.* (1991) Effects of communication skills training on students' diagnostic efficiency. *Med Educ.* **25**: 517–26.

Faden R, Becker C, Lewis C *et al.* (1981) Disclosure of information of patients in medical care. *Med Care.* **19**: 718–33.

Fallowfield L (1993) Giving sad and bad news. *Lancet.* **341**: 476–8.

Fallowfield LJ, Hall A, Maguire GP *et al.* (1990) Psychological outcomes of different treatment policies in women with early breast cancer outside a clinical trial. *BMJ.* **301**: 575–80.

Field D (1995) Education for palliative care: formal education about death and dying and bereavement in UK medical schools in 1983 and 1994. *Med Educ.* **29**: 414–19.

Finlay I and Dallimore D (1991) Your child is dead. *BMJ.* **302**: 1524–5

Francis V, Korsch, B and Morris M (1969) Gaps in doctor–patient communication. *N Engl J Med.* **280**: 535–40.

Frank E, Kupfer DJ and Siegel LR (1995) Alliance not compliance: a philosophy of outpatient care. *J Clin Psychiat.* **56**: 11–17.

Freidson E (1970) *Professional dominance.* Atherton Press, Chicago, IL.

Friedman HS (1979) Non-verbal communication between patient and medical practitioners. *J Soc Issues.* **35**: 82–99.

Gask L, Goldberg D, Lesser AL *et al.* (1988) Improving the psychiatric skills of the general practice trainee: an evaluation of a group training course. *Med Educ.* **22**: 132–8.

Gazda GM, Asbury FR, Balzer FJ *et al.* (1995) *Human relations development: a manual for educators* (5th edn). Allyn and Bacon, Boston, MA.

Gibb JR (1961) Defensive communication. *J Commun.* **3**: 142.

Gick ML (1986) Problem-solving strategies. *Educ Psychologist.* **21**: 99–120.

Goldberg D, Steele JJ, Smith C *et al.* (1983) *Training family practice residents to recognize psychiatric disturbances.* National Institute of Mental Health, Rockville, MD.

Good MJD and Good BJ (1982) Patient requests in primary care clinics. In *Clinically applied anthropology* (eds NJ Crissman and TW Maritzla). D Reidel, Boston, MA.

Greenfield S, Kaplan SH and Ware JE (1985) Expanding patient involvement in care. *Ann Intern Med.* **102**(4): 520–8.

Griffiths F (1995) Women's health concerns. Is the promotion of hormone replacement therapy for prevention important to women? *Fam Prac.* **12**: 54–9.

Grol R, van Beurden W, Binkhorst T *et al.* (1991) Patient education in family practice: the consensus reached by patients, doctors and experts. *Fam Prac.* **8**: 133–9.

Hack TF, Degner LF and Dyck DG (1994) Relationship between preferences for decision control and illness information among women with breast cancer. *Soc Sci Med.* **39**: 279–89.

Hadlow J and Pitts M (1991) The understanding of common terms by doctors, nurses and patients. *Soc Sci Med.* **32**: 193–6.

Hall JA, Roter DL and Rand CS (1981) Communication of affect between patient and physician. *J Health Soc Behav.* **22**: 18–30.

Hall JA, Roter DL and Katz NR (1987) Task versus socioeconomic behaviour in physicians. *Med Care.* **25**: 399–412.

Hall JA, Roter DL and Katz NR (1988) Meta-analysis of correlates of provider behaviour in medical encounters. *Med Care.* **26**: 657–75.

Hall JA, Harrigan JA and Rosenthal R (1995) Non-verbal behaviour in clinician–patient interaction. *Appl Prevent Psychol.* **4**: 21–35.

Hampton JR, Harrison MJG, Mitchell JRA *et al.* (1975) Relative contributions of history-taking, physical examination and laboratory investigation to diagnosis and management of medical out-patients. *BMJ.* **2**: 486–9.

Harrigan JA, Oxman TE and Rosenthal R (1985) Rapport expressed through non-verbal behaviour. *J Non-verbal Behav.* **9**: 95–110.

Haug M and Lavin B (1983) *Consumerism in medicine: challenging physician authority.* Sage Publications, Beverly Hills, CA.

Haynes RB, Taylor DW and Sackett DL (1979) *Compliance in health care.* Johns Hopkins University Press, Baltimore, MD.

Heath C (1984) Participation in the medical consultation: the coordination of verbal and non-verbal behaviour between the doctor and the patient. *Sociol Health and Illness.* **6**: 311–38.

Helman CG (1978) Feed a cold, starve a fever – folk models of infection in an English suburban community and their relation to medical treatment. *Culture, Med Psychiat.* **2**: 107–37.

Helman CG (1981) Disease versus illness in general practice. *JRCGP.* **31**: 548–52.

Henbest RJ and Stewart M (1990a) Patient-centredness in the consultation. 1. A method of measurement. *Fam Prac.* **6**: 249–53.

Henbest RJ and Stewart M (1990*b*) Patient-centredness in the consultation. 2. Does it really make a difference? *Fam Prac.* **7**: 28–33.

Herman JM (1985) The use of patients' preferences in family practice. *J Fam Prac.* **20**: 153–6.

Heron J (1975) *A six-category intervention analysis.* Human Potential Research Project, University of Surrey.

Hope S and Rees MCP (1995) Why do British women start and stop hormone replacement therapy? *J Br Menopausal Society.* **1**(2): 26–8.

Horder J, Byrne P, Freeling P *et al.* (1972) *The future general practitioner: learning and teaching.* Royal College of General Practitioners, London.

Hulka BS (1979) Patient–clinician interaction. In *Compliance in health care* (eds RB Haynes, DW Taylor and DL Sackett). Johns Hopkins University Press, Baltimore, MD.

Inui TS, Yourtee EL and Williamson JW (1976) Improved outcomes in hypertension after physician tutorials. *Ann Intern Med.* **84**: 646–51.

Johnson TM, Hardt EJ and Kleinman A (1995) Cultural factors. In *The medical interview: clinical care, education and research* (eds M Lipkin *et al.*). Springer-Verlag, New York.

Joos SK, Hickam DH and Borders LM (1993) Patients' desires and satisfaction in general medical clinics. *Public Health Reports.* **108**: 751–9.

Joos SK, Hickam DH, Gordon GH *et al.* (1996) Effects of a physician communication intervention on patient care outcomes. *J Gen Intern Med.* **11**: 147–55.

Kaplan SH, Greenfield S and Ware JE (1989) Assessing the effects of physician–patient interactions on the outcomes of chronic disease. *Med Care.* **27**: S110–27.

Kaplan SH, Greenfield S, Gandek B *et al.* (1996) Characteristics of physicians with participatory decision-making styles. *Ann Intern Med.* **124**: 497–504.

Kassirer JP (1983) Teaching clinical medicine by iterative hypothesis testing. *N Engl J Med.* **309**: 921–3.

Kassirer JP and Gorry GA (1978) Clinical problem-solving: a behavioural analysis. *Ann Intern Med.* **89**: 893–900.

Keller VF and Carroll JG (1994) A new model for physician–patient communication. *Patient Educ Couns.* **23**: 131–40.

Keller V and Kemp-White M (1997) *Choice and changes: clinical influence and Patient Action workshop workbook.* Bayer Institute for Health Communication, West Haven, CT.

Kessel N (1979) Reassurance. *Lancet.* **1**: 1128–33.

Kindelan K and Kent G (1987) Concordance between patients' information preferences and general practitioners' perceptions. *Psychology and Health.* **1**: 399–409.

Kleinman A, Eisenberg L and Good B (1978) Culture, illness and care: clinical lessons from anthropologic and cross-cultural research. *Ann Intern Med.* **88**: 251–8.

Koch R (1971) The teacher and non-verbal communication. *Theory Prac.* **10**: 231.

Korsch BM, Gozzi EK and Francis V (1968) Gaps in doctor–patient communication. *Pediatrics.* **42**: 855–71.

Kravitz RL, Cope DW, Bhrany V *et al.* (1994) Internal medical patients' expectations for care during office visits. *J Gen Intern Med.* **9**: 75–81.

Kupst M, Dresser K, Schulman JL *et al.* (1975) Evaluation of methods to improve communication in the physician–patient relationship. *Am J Orthopsychiat.* **45**: 420.

Kurtz SM (1983) *A format for teaching information-giving skills to health professionals.* Education Resources Information Centre (ERIC) 222928.

Kurtz SM (1989) Curriculum structuring to enhance communication skills development. In *Communicating with medical patients* (eds M Stewart and D Roter). Sage Publications, Newbury Park, CA.

Kurtz SM and Silverman JD (1996) The Calgary–Cambridge observation guides: an aid to defining the curriculum and organizing the teaching in communication training programmes. *Med Educ.* **30**: 83–9.

Larsen KM and Smith CK (1981) Assessment of non-verbal communication in the patient–physician interview. *J Fam Prac.* **12**: 481–8.

Lazare A, Eisenthal S and Wasserman L (1975) The customer approach to patienthood: attending to patient requests in a walk-in clinic. *Arch Gen Psychiat.* **32**: 553–8.

Leopold N, Cooper J and Clancy C (1996) Sustained partnership in primary care. *J Fam Prac.* **2**: 129–37.

Levenstein JH, Belle Brown J, Weston WW *et al.* (1989) Patient-centred clinical interviewing. In *Communicating with medical patients* (eds M Stewart and D Roter). Sage Publications, Newbury Park, CA.

Levinson W, Stiles WB, Inui TS *et al.* (1993) Physician frustration in communicating with patients. *Med Care.* **31**(4): 285–95.

Levinson W and Roter D (1995) Physicians' psychosocial beliefs correlate with their patient communication skills. *J Gen Intern Med.* **10**: 375–9.

Levinson W, Roter DL, Mullooly JP *et al.* (1997) The relationship with malpractice claims among primary care physicians and surgeons. *JAMA.* **277**: 553–9.

Ley P (1988) *Communication with patients: improving satisfaction and compliance.* Croom Helm, London.

Lipkin M Jr (1987) The medical interview and related skills. In *The office practice of medicine* (ed WT Branch), pp. 1287–1306. WB Saunders and Co., Philadelphia.

Lipkin M Jr, Putnam SM and Lazare A (1995) *The medical interview.* Springer-Verlag, New York.

Little P, Williamson I, Warner G *et al.* (1997) Open randomised trial of prescribing strategies in managing sore throat. *BMJ.* **314**: 722–7.

McCroskey JC, Larson CE and Knapp ML (1971) *An introduction to interpersonal communication.* Prentice-Hall, Englewood Cliffs, NJ.

McKinlay JB (1975) Who is really ignorant – physician or patient? *J Health Soc Behav.* **16**: 3–11.

Macleod J (1964) *Clinical examination.* Churchill Livingstone, Edinburgh.

McWhinney I (1989) The need for a transformed clinical method. In *Communicating with medical patients* (eds M Stewart and D Roter). Sage Publications, Newbury Park, CA.

Maguire P and Faulkner A (1988) Communicate with cancer patients. 1. Handling bad news and difficult questions. *BMJ.* **297**: 907–9.

Maguire P and Rutter D (1976) History-taking for medical students. 1. Deficiencies in performance. *Lancet.* **2**: 556–8.

Maguire P, Fairbairn S and Fletcher C (1986) Consultation skills of young doctors. 1. Benefits of feedback training in interviewing as students persist. *BMJ.* **292**: 1573–6.

Maguire P, Fairbairn S and Fletcher C (1986) Consultation skills of young doctors. II. Most young doctors are bad at giving information. *BMJ*. **292**: 1576–8.

Maguire P, Faulkner A, Booth K *et al.* (1996) Helping cancer patients disclose their concern. *Eur J Cancer*. **32A**: 78–81.

Maiman LA, Becker MH, Liptak GS *et al.* (1988) Improving pediatricians' compliance-enhancing practices: a randomized trial. *Am J Dis Child*. **142**: 773–9.

Makoul G, Arnston P and Scofield T (1995) Health promotion in primary care: physician–patient communication and decision about prescription medications. *Soc Sci Med*. **41**: 1241–54.

Mandin H, Jones A, Woloshuk W *et al.* (1997) Helping students learn to think like experts when solving clinical problems. *Acad Med*. **72**: 173–9.

Maynard DW (1990) Bearing bad news. *Med Encounter*. **7**: 2–3.

Mazzullo JM, Lasagna L and Griner PF (1974) Variations in interpretation of prescription instructions. *JAMA*. **227**: 929–31.

Mehrabian A (1972) *Non-verbal communication*. Aldine Atherton, Chicago, IL.

Mehrabian A and Ksionsky S (1974) *A theory of affiliation*. Lexington Books, DC Health and Co., Lexington, MA.

Meichenbaum D and Turk DC (1987) *Facilitating treatment adherence: a practitioner's guidebook*. Plenum Press, New York.

Miller SM and Mangan CE (1983) Interacting effects of information and coping styles in adapting to gynaecological stress: should the doctor tell all? *J Personality and Soc Psychol*. **45**: 223–36.

Miller WR (1983) Motivational interviewing with problem drinkers. *Behavioural Psychotherapy*. **11**: 147–52.

Miller WR and Rollnick S (1991) *Motivational interviewing: preparing people to change addictive behavior*. Guilford Press, New York.

Mischler EG (1984) *The discourse of medicine: dialectics of medical interviews*. Ablex, Norwood, NJ.

Mumford E, Schlesinger HJ and Glass GV (1982) The effects of psychological intervention on recovery from surgery and heart attacks: an analysis of the literature. *AJPH*. **72**: 141–51.

Myerscough PR (1992) *Talking with patients*. Oxford University Press, Oxford.

Neighbour R (1987) *The inner consultation: how to develop an effective and intuitive consulting style*. MTP Press, Lancaster.

Novack DH, Dube C and Goldstein MG (1992) Teaching medical interviewing: a basic course on interviewing and the physician–patient relationship. *Arch Intern Med*. **152**: 1814–20.

Orth JE, Stiles WB, Scherwitz L *et al.* (1987) Patient exposition and provider explanation in routine interviews and hypertensive patients' blood pressure control. *Health Psychol*. **6**: 29–42.

Parsons T (1951) *The social system*. Free Press, New York.

Pendleton D, Schofield T, Tate P *et al.* (1984) *The consultation: an approach to learning and teaching*. Oxford University Press, Oxford.

Peppiatt R (1992) Eliciting patients' views of the cause of their problem: a practical strategy for GPs. *Fam Prac*. **9**: 295–8.

Peterson MC, Holbrook J, VonHales D et al. (1992) Contributions of the history, physical examination and laboratory investigation in making medical diagnoses. *West J Med.* **156**: 163–5.

Pinder R (1990) *The management of chronic disease: patient and doctor perspectives on Parkinson's disease.* Macmillan Press, London.

Platt FW and McMath JC (1979) Clinical hypocompetence: the interview. *Ann Intern Med.* **91**: 898–902.

Platt FW and Keller VF (1994) Empathic communication: a teachable and learnable skill. *J Gen Intern Med.* **9**: 222–6.

Poole AD and Sanson-Fisher RW (1979) Understanding the patient: a neglected aspect of medical education. *Soc Sci Med.* **13A**: 37.

Priest V and Speller V (1991) *The risk factor management manual.* Radcliffe Medical Press, Oxford.

Prochaska JO and DiClemente CC (1986) Towards a comprehensive model of change. In *Treating addictive behaviors* (eds R Miller and N Heather). Plenum Press, New York.

Putnam SM, Stiles WB, Jacob, MC et al. (1988) Teaching the medical interview: an intervention study. *J Gen Intern Med.* **3**: 38–47.

Quill TE (1983) Partnerships in patient care: a contractual approach. *Ann Intern Med.* **98**: 228–34.

Reilly S and Muzarkara B (1978) *Mixed message resolution by disturbed adults and children.* Behavioral Sciences Clinical Research Center, Philadelphia State Hospital. A paper presented at the International Communication Association Annual Conference, Chicago, IL.

Riccardi VM and Kurtz SM (1983) *Communication and counselling in health care.* Charles C Thomas, Springfield, IL.

Rogers CR (1980) *A way of being.* Houghton Mifflin, Boston, MA.

Rost KM, Flavin KS, Cole K et al. (1991) Change in metabolic control and functional status after hospitalisation. *Diabetes Care.* **14**: 881–9.

Roter DL (1977) Patient participation in the patient–provider interaction: the effects of patient question-asking on the quality of interaction, satisfaction and compliance. *Health Education Monographs.* **5**: 281–315.

Roter DL and Hall JA (1987) Physicians' interviewing styles and medical information obtained from patients. *J Gen Intern Med.* **2**: 325–9.

Roter DL and Hall JA (1992) *Doctors talking with patients, patients talking with doctors.* Auburn House, Westport, CT.

Roter DL, Hall JA, Kern DE et al. (1995) Improving physicians' interviewing skills and reducing patients' emotional distress. *Arch Intern Med.* **155**: 1877–84.

Rowe MB (1986) Wait time: slowing down may be a way of speeding up. *J Teacher Educ.* **37**: 43–50.

Rutter M and Cox A (1981) Psychiatric interviewing techniques. I. Methods and measures. *Br J Psychiat.* **138**: 273–82.

Sandler G (1980) The importance of the history in the medical clinic and the cost of unnecessary tests. *Am Heart J.* **100**: 928–31.

Sanson-Fisher RW (1981) *Personal communication.* Faculty of Medicine. University of Newcastle, New South Wales, Australia.

Sanson-Fisher RW (1992) *How to break bad news to cancer patients. An interactional skills manual for interns.* The Professional Education and Training Committee of the New South Wales Cancer Council and the Postgraduate Medical Council of NSW Australia, Kings Cross, NSW, Australia.

Sanson-Fisher RW, Redman S, Walsh R *et al.* (1991) Training medical practitioners in information transfer skills: the new challenge. *Med Educ.* **25**: 322–33.

Schulman BA (1979) Active patient orientation and outcomes in hypertensive treatment. *Med Care.* **17**: 267–81.

Simpson M, Buckman R, Stewart M *et al.* (1991) Doctor–patient communication: the Toronto consensus statement. *BMJ.* **303**: 1385–7.

Slack WV (1977) The patient's right to decide. *Lancet.* **July 30**: 240.

Smith RC and Hoppe RB (1991) The patient's story: integrating the patient and physician-centred approaches to interviewing. *Ann Intern Med.* **115**: 471–7.

Sommer R (1971) Social parameters in naturalistic health research. In *Behavior and environment – the use of space by animals and men* (ed A Esser). Plenum Press, New York.

Spiegel D, Bloom KR, Kraemer HC *et al.* (1989) Effect of psychological treatment on survival of patients with metatstatic breast cancer. *Lancet.* **2**: 888–91.

Spiro H (1992) What is empathy and can it be taught? *Ann Intern Med.* **16**: 843–6.

Starfield B, Wray C, Hess K *et al.* (1981) The influence of patient–practitioner agreement on outcome of care. *AJPH.* **71**: 127–31.

Steptoe A, Sutcliffe I, Allen B *et al.* (1991) Satisfacton with communication, medical knowledge and coping styles in patients with metastatic cancer. *Soc Sci Med.* **32**: 627–32.

Stewart MA (1984) What is a successful doctor–patient interview? A study of interactions and outcomes. *Soc Sci Med.* **19**: 167–75.

Stewart MA (1985) *Comparison of two methods of analysing doctor–patient communication.* Paper presented at the North American Primary Care Research Group, Seattle.

Stewart MA (1995) Effective physician–patient communication and health outcomes: a review. *Can Med Assoc J.* **152**: 1423–33.

Stewart MA, McWhinney IR and Buck CW (1979) The doctor–patient relationship and its effect upon outcome. *JRCGP.* **29**: 77–82.

Stewart MA and Roter D (eds) (1989) *Communicating with medical patients.* Sage Publications, Newbury Park, CA.

Stewart MA, Belle Brown J, Wayne Weston W *et al.* (1995) *Patient–centred medicine: transforming the clinical method.* Sage, Thousand Oaks, CA.

Stewart MA, Belle Brown J, Donner A *et al.* (1997) *The impact of patient-centred care on patient outcomes in family practice.* Research report, Thames Valley Family Practice Research Unit, Ontario.

Stiles WB, Putnam SM, James SA *et al.* (1979) Dimensions of patient and physician roles in medical screening interviews. *Soc Sci Med.* **13A**: 335–41.

Stillman PL, Sabars DL and Redfield DL (1976) Use of paraprofessionals to teach interviewing skills. *Pediatrics.* **57**: 769–74.

Stimson GV and Webb B (1975) *Going to see the doctor.* Routledge and Kegan Paul, London.

Strull WM, Lo B and Charles G (1984) Do patients want to participate in medical decision-making? *JAMA*. **252**: 2990–4.

Sutherland HJ, Llewellyn-Thomas HA and Lockwood GA (1989) Cancer patients: their desire for information and participation in treatment decisions. *J R Soc Med*. **82**: 260.

Svarstad BL (1974) *The doctor–patient encounter: an observational study of communication and outcome*. Doctoral dissertation, University of Wisconsin, Madison.

Tait I (1979) *The history and function of clinical records*. Unpublished MD dissertation thesis, University of Cambridge.

Tate P (1997) *The doctor's communication handbook* (2nd edn). Radcliffe Medical Press, Oxford.

The Headache Study Group of The University of Western Ontario (1986) Predictors of outcome in headache patients presenting at family physicians – a one-year prospective study. *Headache J*. **26**: 285–94,

Truax CB and Carkhuff RR (1967) *Towards effective counselling and psychotherapy*. Aldine, Chicago, IL.

Tuckett D, Boulton M, Olson C *et al.* (1985) *Meetings between experts: an approach to sharing ideas in medical consultations*. Tavistock, London.

van Bilsen HP and van Emst AJ (1989) Motivating heroin-users for change. In *Treating drug abusers* (ed GA Bennett). Routledge, London.

van Thiel J, Kraan HF and van der Vleuten CPM (1991) Reliability and feasibility of measuring medical interviewing skills: the revised Maastricht history–taking and advice checklist. *Med Educ*. **25**: 224–9.

Verderber RF and Verderber KS (1980) *Interact: using interpersonal communication skills*. Wadsworth, Belmont, CA.

Waitzkin H (1984) Doctor–patient communication: clinical implications of social scientific research. *JAMA*. **252**: 2441–6.

Waitzkin H (1985) Information-giving in medical care. *J Health Soc Behav*. **26**: 81–101.

Walton J, Duncan AS, Fletcher CM *et al.* (1980) *Talking with patients, a teaching approach*. Nuffield Provincial Hospitals Trust, London.

Wasserman RC, Inui TS, Barriatua RD *et al.* (1984) Pediatric clinicians' support for parents makes a difference: an outcome-based analysis of clinician–parent interaction. *Pediatrics*. **6**: 1047–53.

Watzlawick P, Beavin J and Jackson D (1967) *Pragmatics of human communication*. WW Norton, New York.

Weinberger M, Greene JY and Mamlin JJ (1981) The impact of clinical encounter events on patient and physician satisfaction. *Soc Sci Med*. **15E**: 239–44.

White J, Levinson W and Roter D (1994) 'Oh, by the way' – the closing moments of the medical interview. *J Gen Intern Med*. **9**: 24–8.

Wissow LS, Roter DL and Wilson MEH (1994) Pediatrician interview style and mothers' disclosure of psychosocial issues. *Pediatrics*. **93**: 289–95.

WHO (1985) *Targets for health for all*. WHO Regional Office for Europe, Copenhagen.

Woolley H, Stein A, Forrest GC *et al.* (1989) Imparting the diagnosis of life-threatening illness in children. *BMJ*. **41**: 1623–6.

Wright LM, Watson WL and Bell JM (1996) *Beliefs: the heart of healing in families and illness*. Basic Books, New York.

Index

acceptance 74, 79
  accepting response 79–81, *94*, 124
  not agreement 81–2
  patients' views *94*, 122
  premature reassurance problem 82
  responding to indirectly expressed feelings
    and emotions 81
  responding to overt feelings and emotions
    80–1
accuracy, goals of medical education 14
acknowledging response *see* acceptance:
    accepting response
adherence, *see* compliance
affect, communicating 75
affiliation and patient satisfaction 85
agenda-eliciting and identifying 31–2
agenda setting *19*, 32–3, 131
agreement, acceptance is not 81–2
anthropological studies and disease-illness
    model 57–8
assumptions 21–9, 31, 66–7, 78, 83, 100–1, 116,
    141
attentive listening *see* listening
attitudes xviii, 75
authority, doctors' 85

bad news, breaking 136–41
  key core and issue-specific skills, framework
    138–9
beliefs *44*, 56–8, 62–3, *93*, *94*, 115, 122
breadth
  Calgary–Cambridge observation guide
    5
building the relationship *see* relationship
    building

Calgary–Cambridge observation guide
  function and purpose *5–6*
  structure *6*
    framework *7*
    individual skills *8–11*
    tasks *6–7*
      building the relationship *74*
      closing the session *132*
      explanation and planning *93–4*, *121*, *123*
      gathering information *44*
      initiating the session *19*
categorization *93*, 103
challenging patients 124–6
choices, offers *94*, 121
chunking and checking *93*, 101, 104
clarification *44*, 54–5
clinical competence 1
clinical detachment 72–3
clinical performance 2
clinical skills 1
closed questions *see* questioning style
closing the session 10–11, 129, *132*
  earlier behaviours preventing new problems
    131–2
  elements of
    contracting 133
    end summary 132–3
    final checking 133
    safety-netting 133
  inefficient endings 132
  patients' 'hidden agendas' 131
  objectives 130
  skills *132*
    evidence for 130–3
  summarizing 132–3

co-ordinated approach to communication skills teaching xviii
collaborative approach to planning *see* planning
collaborative partnership 3
comfort
    doctors' self-comfort 19, 20
    patients' physical comfort 19, 20
commitment to plans made *94*, 112–13
competence gap 96, 97
compliance 117
    communication problems 91
    interviewing skills for aiding 114–15
    studies 59–60
conceptual framework 12
concerns *44*, 56–8, 62–3, *94*, 122, 131
confrontation 124–6, *125*
    core skills 16, 135
consultations *see* sessions
consumerism model 116
content skills 4
continuing medical education xviii
contracting 133
    contribution, encourages patients' *93*, 115
convergent questions *see* questioning style: closed questions
cross-cultural studies 57–8
cross-cultural teaching xix, 143
cues
    non-verbal 29, *62*, 74, *93*, 115
    picking up and checking out 61–2
    verbal 29, *62*, *93*, 115
    see also non-verbal communication; verbal communication
cultural background, takes into consideration if negotiating a mutual plan of action *94*, 122
cultural issues, key core and issue-specific skills 141–3
    cross-cultural studies 57–8
    cross-cultural teaching xix

decision making, shared *94*, 120–2
decoding non-verbal cues 78
default model, doctor–patient control 116
depression, key core and issue-specific skills 145–6
developing rapport *74*
    acceptance *see* acceptance

empathy 83
    communicating to patients 84
    statements expressing 86
    understanding patients' predicament and feelings 83
    research evidence 85–6
    support 85
diagnostic-significance of problems in Tuckett *et al.*'s methodology 107
diagrams, visual methods of conveying information *93*, 106
directives, making suggestions rather than *94*, 121
disease, definition and the disease–illness model 38–9
disease–illness model 38, *39*
    disease, definition 38–9
    illness, definition 38–9
    information gathering
        explanation, groundwork for 41–2
        integration 42
        need to explore both doctors' and patients' perspectives 40–2
        planning, groundwork for 41
        relationship building 40–1
        support 40–1
        understanding 40–1
    information giving 108
distortion in communication 67
divergent questions *see* questioning style: open questions
divergent views of doctors and patients 112
doctor-centred closed approach to information gathering 36
doctor–patient relationship 1
    consumerism 116
    default or laissez-faire model of doctor–patient control 116
    models 115–16
    mutuality 116
    paternalistic 116
    traditional view
        emotional nature of illness 96, 97
        modern research misinterpretation 97–8
        professional authority 96–7
        unbridgeable competence gap 96, 97
dynamism 32
    principles that demonstrate effective communication *15*

echoing 52
effects on life 44, 64
effective communication, goals of medical
       communication 2, *14*
efficiency 14, *see* goals of medical education
emotions
   communicating 75
   exploring 131
   illness, emotional nature of 96, 97
   physicians showing 132
   responding to 80–1
empathy 74, 83
   communicating to patients 84
   poor skills in 72
   research evidence that expressing is effective
      86
   understanding patients' predicament and
      feelings 83
encoding 77, 78
encouragement 44, 51–2, 93, *94*, 115, 122
endings, *see* closure
end summary 65, 132–3
establishing initial rapport *see* initiating the
     session
evidence-based approach xvii, 3
evidence research for skills
   amount of information should be given 95
   attentive listening 26–7
   building the relationship, problems 85–6
   collaborative approach to 118–20
   endings 130–1
   exploring patient's perspective 41, 57–61
   explanation and planning, problems in 90–2
   facilitation 53
   gathering information, problems in 35–6
   identifying why the person came, problems in
     23
   individual skills of *Calgary–Cambridge guides*
     3, 6, 13
   information, more is helpful 99–100
    do all patients want more? 100
   non-verbal communication 76–7
    notes, use of 78–9
   patient understanding 106–15
   rapport-building, of 85–6
   recall of information 97–8, 103–6
   summarizing in 66
expectations *44*, 58–60, 62–3, 114–15
explanation 9–*10*, 82, 89, 93, *94*
   communication problems 89

information given by doctors 90
   language used by doctors 90–1
   recall and understanding 91
   teaching problems 91–2
groundwork for 41–2
information giving
   on action or treatment offered *94*, 123
   amount 95
   clarity 108
   communication problems 89
   correct amount and type *93*, 95–102
   increased amount is helpful 99–100
   patients
     autonomy 99
     desire for more information 100
     influence of 109–10
     involvement 110
     perspective of 107
     recall of information 97–8
     satisfaction 99–100
   prejudices, confirmation of 98
   recall *see* recall
   recent influences on
     changes in medicine 99
     changes in society 98
     patient autonomy 99
     research results 108–13
     shared understanding 111–12
     sharing of views 108
     skills required
       chunking and checking *93*, 101
       offering other information *93*, 102
       patients' prior knowledge, assessing *93*,
        101–2
       timing *93*, 102
     theoretical framework for research
       methodology (Tuckett *et al.*) 107–8
     traditional view of doctor–patient
       relationship
       emotional nature of illness 96, 97
       modern research misinterpretation 97–8
       professional authority 96–7
       unbridgeable competence gap 96, 97
     treatment offered *94*, 123
     understanding 111–12
interactive collaborative process 126–7
investigations and procedures 126
objectives 92
offering opinions *94*, 121–2
options *94*, 121–6

patient commitment 112–13
  outcome measures 108
patient contribution 93, 115
patient recall *see* recall
patient understanding
      see understanding
patients' illness framework 93, 115
patients' perspective, alternative ways of
      exploring 61, *93*, 106–15
shared understanding *93*, 106–15
skills, evidence for *93–4*, 93–115
understanding *see* understanding
exploration of problems 8, 43–56, *see also*
      gathering information
eye contact 29, *74*, 76, 78–9

facial expression *44*, 74
facilitative response 51
  encouragement 51–2
  listening *28*, 51
  paraphrasing *53*
  repetition or echoing 52
  silence 52
  theoretical evidence 53
facilitators xx
  awareness of structure 12
family medicine
  unified approach to teaching
      xviii–xix
feedback *see* summarizing
feelings
  patients' *44*, 63, *64*, 80–1
final checking 132–3
follow-up visits 25
framework of *Calgary–Cambridge observation guide*
      7
functional enquiry 56
funding agencies xx–xxi

gathering information *see* information gathering
general practice
  unified approach to teaching xviii–xix
goals of medical communication *14*
greeting *19*, 20

health outcomes, improvement 3
helical nature of communication *15*, 66
'hidden agendas' of patients 26, 131
history taking *see* information gathering:
      traditional method

ideas *44*, 56–8, 62–3, 131
identifying reasons for consultation 19, 22–33
  patients' ideas, concerns and expectations
      61–3
illness
  definition 38–9
  emotional nature of 96
  framework *see* information gathering: patients'
      perspective
  see also disease–illness model
individuality, skills and 14–16
information
  unequal importance of in Tuckett *et al.*'s
      research 107
information gathering 8–9, 35
  communication problems 35–6
  disease–illness model *see* disease–illness
      model
  distortion in communication 67
  doctor-centred closed approach 36
  history taking *see* traditional method *below*
  objectives 42–3
  patient-centred clinical interviewing *see*
      disease–illness model
  patients' perspective
    discovering 41
    illness framework 61
      effect on life *44*, 64
      feelings 63, *64*
      non-verbal cues 62, *62*
      picking up and checking out cues 61–2
      specific asking 62–3, *63*
      verbal cues *62*
    integration 57–8
    understanding 56–64
    value of exploring, evidence for 56–7
      anthropological and cross-cultural studies
        57–8
      outcome studies 58–9
      patient-centred interviews, length 61
      satisfaction and compliance studies 59–60
      understanding and recall studies 60
  problem exploration 43
    attentive listening *44*, 51
    clarification of patients' story 54
    closed questioning *44*, 54–6
    facilitative response 51
      encouragement 51–2
      paraphrasing 53
      repetition or echoing 52

silence 52
  theoretical evidence 53
functional enquiry *55*, 56
internal summary 54
language 56
open questioning *44*, 50–1, 53
patients' narrative 50–1
questioning style *see* questioning style
skills *44*, 50–6
symptoms, analysis 55–6, *55*
thought sharing 56
questioning style *see* questioning style
sequencing *44*, 70
signposting *44*, 67–8, 68–9
skills *44*
  evidence for 43–70
structure for consultation 65–70
summarizing *see* summarizing
traditional method
  failure to explain everything about patients'
    problems 41
  origins 36–7
  strengths 37
  weaknesses 37–8
transformed clinical method *see* disease–illness
    model
information giving, correct amount and type 93,
    99–102
in closure 131
see also explanation
initiating the session 8, 17, *19*
  common assumptions 23
  communication problems 18
  establishing initial rapport *19, 20*
    greeting and introduction 20–1
    interest, demonstrating *19*, 22
    patients
      name 21
      physical comfort 22
    relationship building, contribution to 22
    respect, demonstrating 22
    role clarification 21
  identifying reasons for consultation 19, 22–3
    agenda setting 32–3
    dynamism 32
    eye contact 29
    follow-up visits 25
    interruption 26–7, 28
    listening *see* listening
    new consultations 24

opening question 24–5
patients
  'hidden agendas' 26
  opening statements 25–30
  verbal and non-verbal cues 29
screening 30–2
objectives 18–19, 25
preparation 19–20
skills, evidence for 19–33
integration
  disease–illness model 42
  patients' perspective 57–8
interaction
  communication as *15*, 33, 66, *93*, 126
  non–verbal 73–4
interactional alignment 114
interactive collaborative process 126–7
interest, demonstrates *19*, 22
internal summary *see* summarizing
interruption 26–7, 28
introduces, self *19*, 20–1
investigations and procedures 126
involving patients *94*, 121, 131
issue-specific skills 16, 135–48
issues, communication xviii, 16, 135–46

labelling important information *93*, 103–4
laissez-faire model 116
language *44*, 56, 90–1, *93*, 105
learners xix
  awareness of structure 12
learning communication skills 2
lifestyle, patients'
  take into consideration if negotiating a mutual
    plan of action *94*, 122
listening
  achievement of more objectives 25
  advantages of 29
  attentive 27–30, 131
  evidence to support 26–7
  facilitative response 28
  non-verbal skills 28–9
  problem exploration 51
  and screening, balance between 31–2
  skills *19*, 27–9, *44*, 50–2
  wait time 27–8

malpractice and medico-legal complaints 33, 53,
    69
medical education administrators xx–xxi

medical interviews *see* sessions
medical politicians xx–xxi
medicine, changes in 99
mental illness 143–5
motivational interviewing 123
mutuality model 116
mutually acceptable plan *94*, 121
mutually understood common ground *15*, 29,
      33, 42, 58, 60, 65–6, 69, 82, 113, 119–20,
      134

name, obtaining patient's *19*, 20–1
narrative *44*, 50–1
negotiating agenda 19, 23, 25
  mutual plan of action *94*, 115–21
negotiating mutual plan of action *see* planning
new consultations
  identifying reasons for consultation 24
non-adherence, *see* non-compliance
non-compliance 91, 117
non-verbal communication 73–4, *74*
  communicating attitudes, emotions and affect
     75
  continuous nature 75
  doctors' behaviour 74
  encoding 77, 78
  eye contact 76, 78–9
  lessons for doctors 77–8
  meaning *75*
  mode 75
  notes and records, use of during consultations
     78–9
  patients' cues 74, 78
  operating at edge of or beyond conscious
     awareness 75
  overriding verbal messages 76
  reinforcement theory of social interaction 76
  research evidence 76–7
  skills 28–9
  synchrony 76
  transmitting own cues 78
  understanding aiding consultations 76
  and verbal communication, differences
     between 74–5
non-verbal cues 29, *62*, *74*, 78, *93*, 115 *see also* cues
notes, use of during consultations *74*, 78–9

objectives
  achievement by listening 25
  closure 130

explanation 92
information gathering 42–3
initiating the session 18–19, 25
nature 18–19
planning 92
relationship building 73
open questions *see* questioning style
open-to-closed cone *see* questioning style
opening question *19*, 24–5
opening statements, patients 25–30
  opinion, offers *7*, *94*, 121–2
  options, in explanation opening *94*, 121–2
orientating statements *see* signposting
outcomes
  communication planning in terms of *15*, 18
  measures 108
  health 3, 58–9, 100, 114–15, 118–19

paraphrasing 44, 53
paternalistic model 116
patient-centred approach 3
patient-centred clinical interviewing *see*
      disease–illness model
patient-centred interviews, length 61
  doctor's understanding 60
patient restatement 105
patients
  autonomy 99
  beliefs *44*, 56–8, *93*, 113, 123
  clarification of story *44*, 54
  commitment 112–13
    outcome measures 108
  compliance *see* compliance
  concerns *44*, 58, 62–3, *93*, 115
  contribution *93*, 115
  desire for more information 100
  feelings 63, *64*, *93*
  'hidden agendas' 26, 131
  illness framework *93*, 115
  influence of on doctors' information giving
     109–10
  involvement *74*, 86, *94*, 110, 121
    checking understanding 87
    providing rationale 87–8
    relationship building *see* relationship
      building
    summarizing 87
    thought sharing 87
  name 21
  narrative 50–1

non-verbal cues 74, 78
opening statements 25–30
perspective of *93*, 106–15
    discovering *see* information gathering
physical comfort 22
prior knowledge, assessing *93*, 101–2
reactions *93*, 115
recall of information 97–8
restatement 105
satisfaction 99–100
    studies 59–60
verbal and non-verbal cues 29
views, obtaining *94*, 113, 123, 124–6
perceptual skills 4
perspective, patients' *93*, 106–15
planning 9–10, 89, *93*, *94*
    collaborative approach
        checking with patients *94*, 121
        choices *94*, 121
        compliance 117
        consumerism model 116
        default model 116
        doctor–patient relationship models 115–16
        laissez-faire model 116
        mutuality 116
        negotiating mutually acceptable plans *94*,
            121
        non-compliance 117
        paternalistic model 116
        patient involvement *94*, 121
        research evidence 118–20
        theoretical evidence 117–18
        theory behind 115–18
        thought sharing *94*, 120–1
    communication problems 89
        patient compliance or adherence 91
        teaching problems 91–2
    disease–illness model groundwork for
        41
    interactive collaborative process 126–7
    investigations and procedures 126
    negotiating mutual plan of action *94*, 121,
        122
        accepting response *94*, 124–6
        challenging patients 124–6
        confrontation 124–6, *125*
        motivational interviewing 123
        options in management and treatment *94*,
            122
        patients' views, obtaining *94*, 123

providing information on action or
    treatment *94*, 123
    stages of change model 123, *124*
objectives 92
offering opinions *94*, 121–2
options *94*, 121–6
shared decision-making *94*, 115–21
skills, evidence for *94*, 115–26
power 85
practitioners
    awareness of structure 12
preceptors *see* facilitators
premature reassurance problem 82
preparation 19–20
preventive measures 107
primacy effect 103–4
principles characterizing effective
    communication *15*
problem list *see* screening
procedures, if discussing *94*, 126
process skills 4
professional authority 96–7
professional distance 85
programme directors xx
protection 95
psycho-social issues 131
psychotic patients, key core and issue-specific
    skills 143–4

questioning style, key core and issue-specific
    skills *44*, 43–5
    closed questions 54–6
        evidence for value of 48–9
        meaning and nature 45
        movement from open questions to 48
        psychotic patients 143
        stab-in-the-dark approach 47
        use 45–6
    open questions 45, 50–1, 53
        advantages 46–8
        diagnostic reasoning, contributing to
            47
        disease and illness framework, exploration
            of 47–8
        doctors' listening and thinking time 47
        encouraging patients 46–7
        evidence for value of 48–9
        meaning and nature 45
        movement to closed questions from 48
        patient participation encouragement 48

psychotic patients 143
use 45–6
open-to-closed cone 45–6
psychotic patients 143

rapport
initiating *19*, 20–2
developing *74*, 83–6
see also developing rapport; initiating the
session
rationale, reveals
for opinion 94, 122
for non-sequiturs or examination 74
reactions, elicits patients' *93*, 115, *94*, 122
reasons, identifying for the consultation *19*,
22–33
reassurance, premature 82, 93
recall
aiding accuracy *93*, 102–6
categorization *93*, 103
chunking and checking *93*, 104
communication problems 91
labelling important information 103–4
language *93*, 105
not necessarily implying understanding 107
outcome measures 108
patient restatement 105
repetition *93*, 104–5
research 103–6
primacy effect 103–4
signposting *93*, 103
specific explanation or advice *93*, 105–6
studies 60, 97–8
understanding 93
visual methods of conveying information *93*,
106
records, use of during consultations *74*, 78–9
reinforcement theory of social interaction 76
relationship building 9, 71–2
communication problems 72–3
developing rapport *see* developing rapport
disease–illness model 40–1
empathy *see* empathy
initial rapport contributing to 22
non-verbal communication *see* non-verbal
communication
objectives 73
patient involvement *74*, 86
checking understanding 87
providing rationale 87–8

summarizing 87
thought sharing 87
skills *74*
evidence for 73–88
uncertainty reduction 86
verbal communication *see* verbal
communication
repetition 52, *93*, 104–5
residency, co-ordinated approach to teaching xviii
respect, demonstrates *19*, 20–2
reviews (follow-up visits) 25
role clarification 21

safety-netting 133
satisfaction
doctor 3
patient *see* patients
screening 30–2
sequencing *44*, 70
significance of problems 7, 121–2
sessions
closing *see* closure
differing contexts 17
effectiveness improvement 2
initiating *see* initiating the session
structure 6–7, 65–70
shared decision-making *94*, 115–21
shares thoughts, ideas and dilemmas *94*, 120–1
shut down 138, 140
signposting *44*, 67–8, 68–9, *93*, 103
signposting intent, in confrontation 125
silence 52
skills
Calgary–Cambridge observation guide 5
clinical, core 1
closure 130–3, *132*
content skills 4
core xviii, 16, 135
curriculum, choice for 12–13
communication principles underlying 14
defining broad types 4
in explanation *93–4*, 93–115
and individuality 14–16
information gathering 43–70, *44*
information giving *93*, 101–2
initiating the session 19–33
issue-specific 16
relating to core skills 135–48
overall curriculum of 5
perceptual skills 4

planning *94*, 115–26
problem exploration 50–6
process skills 4
relationship building 73–88, *74*
validation, research and theoretical bases 13
skills-based approach xviii
social interaction, reinforcement theory of 76
society, changes in 98
specialist medicine, unified approach to teaching
xviii–xix
stages of change model 123, *124*
starting point *93*, 101–2
status 85
structure
Calgary–Cambridge observation guide 5
need for 12
providing 65–70
students *see* learners
suggestions, involving patients by making *94*,
121
encouraging patients to contribute *94*, 121
suicidal risk, assessing 145–6
summarizing 87, 103, 132–3
closures 132
end summary 65, *132*
evidence for value of 66–8
internal summaries 44, 54, 65
key skills 65–6, 68
nature of 65
and signposting 69, *93*
support 74, 85, *94*, 122
disease–illness model 40–1
supportive response *see* acceptance: accepting
response
supportiveness, goals of medical education *14*
symptoms, analysis 55–6, *55*

teaching 2
thoughts *44*, 131
thought sharing 56, 74, 87, *94*, 120–1
time 61
time framing *44*
trainers *see* facilitators
transformed clinical method *see* disease–illness
model
treatment action in Tuckett *et al.*'s methodology
107
treatment offered, provides information on *94*,
122
'two parallel monologues' 50

uncertainty reduction *15*, 29, 31, 33, 69, 86–7,
120, 134
undergraduate education, co-ordinated approach
to teaching xviii
understanding
aiding *93*, 102–6
checking 87
communication problems 90–1
diagnostic-significance of problems 107
disease–illness model 40–1
divergent views 112
eliciting beliefs, reactions and concerns 115
implication of problems or treatment 107
information giving *93*, 111–12
non-verbal cues *93*, 115
outcome measures 108
preventive measures 107
recall not necessarily implying commitment
107
research 106–13
shared *93*, 106–15
studies 60
treatment action in Tuckett *et al.*'s
methodology 107
unequal importance of information in Tuckett
et al.'s methodology 107
verbal cues *93*, 115
unified approach
cross-cultural teaching xix
family medicine xviii–xix
international teaching xix
specialist medicine xviii–xix

validity
Calgary–Cambridge observation guide 5, 13
verbal communication
communicating discrete pieces of information
75
mode 75
and non-verbal communication, differences
between 74–5
overridden by non-verbal messages 76
voluntary control 75
verbal cues 29, 62, 74, *93*, 115 *see also* cues
views, obtains patients' *94*, 122
visual methods of conveying information
93, 106

wait time 27–8, 52
warning shot 138, 140

Author Index

Arborelius and Bremberg (1992) 60, 114
Argyle (1975) 75

Baker (1955) 15
Barrows and Tamblyn (1981) 47
Barsevich and Johnson (1990) 100
Barsky (1981) 26, 131
Bass and Cohen (1982) 62, 114
Becker (1974) 117
Beckman and Frankel (1984) 18, 23, 26, 27, 28,
        48, 52, 131
Beckman et al. (1985) 26
Beisecker and Beisecker (1990) 95, 109, 120
Benson and Britten (1996) 140
Berg et al. (1993) 91
Bertakis (1977) 97, 100, 105
Bertakis et al. (1991) 85
Blacklock (1977) 41
Blanchard et al. (1988) 120
Boreham and Gibson (1978) 90, 109, 122
Bouhris et al. (1989) 97
Bradshaw et al. (1975) 105
Briggs and Banahan (1979) 79, 80
Brod et al. (1986) 137
Brody (1980) 117
Brody and Miller (1986) 58
Brody et al. (1989) 118
Broyles et al. (1992) 100
Buckman (1994) 99, 137, 139
Buller and Buller (1987) 85
Burack and Carpenter (1983) 18
Butler et al. (1996) 91, 117, 123
Butow et al. (1994) 119
Byrne and Long (1976) 18, 26, 35, 43, 73, 92, 130

Campion et al. (1992) 38
Carroll and Monroe (1979) 6
Cassata (1978) 6, 33, 70
Cassell (1985) 37, 40
Cassileth et al. (1980) 95, 120
Chugh et al. (1994) 57
Chugh et al. (1993) 16, 142
Coambs et al. (1995) 91, 117
Cohen-Cole (1991) 6, 19, 31, 43, 73, 92, 130
Cox (1989) 49, 61
Cox et al. (1981a) 49, 61, 66

Cox et al. (1981b) 49, 61
Cox et al. (1989) 143
Cushing and Jones (1995) 137

Dance (1967) 15
Dance and Larson (1972) 15, 66, 126
Davies (1997) 143
Deber (1994) 100, 116, 118
Deber et al. (1996) 120
Degner et al. (1997) 120
DeVito (1988) 76
Deyo and Diehl (1986) 100
DiMatteo et al. (1980) 75, 77
DiMatteo et al. (1986) 77
Dye and DiMatteo (1995) 117, 123

Egan (1990) 27, 53, 85
Egbert et al. (1964) 100
Eisenthal and Lazare (1976) 59, 60, 114
Eisenthal et al. (1979) 59, 117, 118
Eisenthal et al. (1990) 59
Ekman et al. (1972) 75
Eleftheriadou (1996) 142, 143
Ely et al. (1995) 20
Ende et al. (1989) 120
Evans et al. (1991) 38

Faden et al. (1981) 95
Fallowfield (1993) 141
Fallowfield et al. (1990) 119
Field (1995) 136
Finlay and Dallimore (1991) 136
Frances et al. (1969) 59
Frank et al. (1995) 117
Freidson (1970) 96
Friedman (1979) 74

Gask et al. (1988) 16
Gazda et al. (1995) 29, 78, 83
Gibb (1961) 80
Gick (1986) 47
Goldberg et al. (1983) 46, 49, 77
Good and Good (1982) 23
Greenfield et al. (1985) 23
Griffiths (1995) 123
Grol et al. (1991) 106

Hack *et al.* (1994) 120
Hadlow and Pitts (1991) 105
Hall *et al.* (1981) 77, 119
Hall *et al.* (1987) 77
Hall *et al.* (1988) 86, 99
Hall *et al.* (1995) 74, 78
Hampton *et al.* (1975) 35
Harrigan *et al.* (1985) 76
Haug and Lavin (1983) 116
Haynes *et al.* (1979) 91
Headache Study Group of the University of
        Western Ontario (1986) 58
Heath (1984) 78, 79
Helman (1978) 102, 107
Helman (1981) 122
Henbest and Stewart (1990*a*) 53, 60
Henbest and Stewart (1990*b*) 53, 60
Herman (1985) 117
Heron (1975) 126
Hope and Rees (1995) 123
Horder *et al.* (1972) 98
Hulka (1979) 97

Inui *et al.* (1976) 114

Johnson *et al.* (1995) 141–2
Joos *et al.* (1993) 59
Joos *et al.* (1996) 33

Kaplan *et al.* (1989) 77, 100, 115, 118, 119
Kaplan *et al.* (1996) 118, 119
Kassirer (1983) 35
Kassirer and Gorry (1978) 47
Keller and Carroll (1994) 19, 38, 43, 73, 92, 130
Keller and Kemp White (1997) 123
Kessel (1979) 82
Kindelan and Kent (1987) 90, 106, 122
Kleinman *et al.* (1978) 36, 40, 57
Koch (1971) 29, 76
Korsch *et al.* (1968) 31, 59, 72, 90
Kravitz *et al.* (1994) 59
Kupst *et al.* (1975) 105
Kurtz (1989) 5, 6
Kurtz and Silverman (1996) 5

Larsen and Smith (1981) 77
Lazare *et al.* (1975) 59
Leopold *et al.* (1996) 72
Levinson and Roter (1995) 61
Levinson *et al.* (1993) 72

Levinson *et al.* (1997) 33, 53, 69
Ley (1988) 91, 97, 98, 103–6, 108, 109, 111
Lipkin (1987) 31
Little *et al.* (1997) 60

McCroskey *et al.* (1971) 29, 76
McKinlay (1975) 90
Macleod (1964) 55
McWhinney (1989) 35, 36, 38
Maguire and Faulkner (1988) 16, 137, 139
Maguire and Rutter (1976) 21, 36
Maguire *et al.* (1986) 6, 16, 89, 91
Maguire *et al.* (1996) 49, 61, 66
Maiman *et al.* (1988) 115
Makoul *et al.* (1995) 90
Mandin *et al.* (1997) 47
Maynard (1990) 114
Mazzullo *et al.* (1974) 105
Mehrabian (1972) 75
Mehrabian and Ksionsky (1974) 31, 76
Meichenbaum and Turk (1987) 91, 117
Miller (1983) 123
Miller and Mangan (1983) 100
Miller and Rollnick (1991) 123
Mischler (1984) 38, 40, 50
Mumford *et al.* (1982) 100
Myerscough (1992) 142

Neighbour (1987) 19, 43, 66, 73, 92, 130, 133
Novack *et al.* (1992) 6

Orth *et al.* (1987) 58

Parsons (1951) 96
Pendleton *et al.* (1984) 19, 43, 73, 92, 130
Peppiatt (1992) 60
Peterson *et al.* (1992) 35
Pinder (1990) 95, 100
Platt and Keller (1994) 83, 84
Platt and McMath (1979) 36
Poole and Sanson-Fisher (1979) 72, 84
Priest and Speller (1991) 123
Prochaska and DiClemente (1986) 123
Putnam *et al.* (1988) 27

Quill (1983) 117

Reilly and Muzarkara (1978) 76
Riccardi and Kurtz (1983) 5, 6, 14, 31
Rogers (1980) 53, 85

Rost *et al.* (1991) 119
Roter (1977) 109, 110, 119
Roter and Hall (1987) 48
Roter and Hall (1992) 115
Roter *et al.* (1995) 59, 61
Rowe (1986) 28, 52
Rutter and Cox (1981) 49, 61

Sandler (1980) 35
Sanson-Fisher (1981) 6
Sanson-Fisher (1992) 137
Sanson-Fisher *et al.* (1991) 6, 16, 89, 92
Schulman (1979) 118
Simpson *et al.* (1991) xix
Slack (1977) 117
Smith and Hoppe (1991) 40
Sommer (1971) 22
Spiegel *et al.* (1989) 86
Spiro (1992) 83
Starfield *et al.* (1981) 18, 23, 114
Steptoe *et al.* (1991) 100
Stewart (1984) 60
Stewart (1985) 61
Stewart (1995) 100, 119
Stewart and Roter (1989) xvii, xix, 39
Stewart *et al.* (1979) 18
Stewart *et al.* (1995) 38
Stewart *et al.* (1997) 41, 117, 119, 133
Stiles *et al.* (1979) 48, 100

Stillman *et al.* (1976) 6
Stimson and Webb (1975) 109
Strull *et al.* (1984) 120
Sutherland *et al.* (1989) 120
Svarstad (1974) 90, 109, 111, 119, 122

Tait (1979) 37
Tate (1997) 123
Truax and Carkhuff (1967) 84
Tuckett *et al.* (1985) 6, 29, 36, 41, 58, 60, 61, 62, 97, 98, 100, 104, 106–13, 119, 122, 136

van Bilson and van Emst (1989) 123
van Thiel *et al* (1991) 6
Verderber and Verderber (1980) 74

Waitzkin (1984) 90, 95
Waitzkin (1985) 100
Walton *et al.* (1980) 91
Wasserman *et al.* (1984) 23, 82, 86
Watzlawick *et al.* (1967) 75
Weinberger *et al.* (1981) 77
White *et al.* (1994) 130, 131, 132
WHO (1985) 123
Wissow *et al.* (1994) 27, 86
Woolley *et al.* (1989) 141
Wright *et al.* (1996) 58